# PITUITARY ADENOMAS

Edited by **Vafa Rahimi-Movaghar**

**Pituitary Adenomas**
Edited by Vafa Rahimi-Movaghar

**Published by InTech**
Janeza Trdine 9, 51000 Rijeka, Croatia



**Publishing Process Manager** Maja Bozicevic

**Technical Editor** Teodora Smiljanic

**Cover Designer** InTech Design Team

Additional hard copies can be obtained from orders@intechopen.com

Pituitary Adenomas, Edited by Vafa Rahimi-Movaghar
p. cm.
ISBN 978-953-51-0041-6

For EU product safety concerns:
IN TECH d.o.o., Prolaz Marije Krucifikse Kozulić 3, 51000 Rijeka, Croatia,
info@intechopen.com or visit our website at intechopen.com.

# Meet the editor

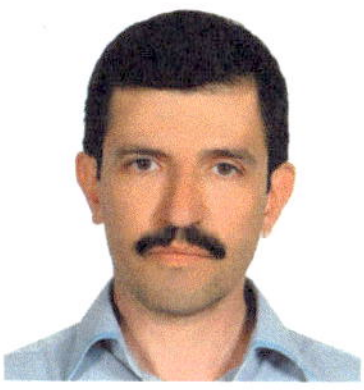

Professor Vafa Rahimi-Movaghar was Neurosurgeon-in-Chief at Khatam-ol-anbia Hospital of Zahedan University Medical Sciences in Iran from 1994 to 2006 and then moved to the Sina Trauma & Surgery Research Center in Tehran University of Medical Sciences. Since 2010 he is Vice-Chairman of the research centre. Since January 2012, he has started to be the guide for PhD by research in Neurotrauma. He has written in neurosurgical topics, with over 100 publications; 61 in SCOPUS and EMBASE; 59 in PUBMED, 54 of them in ISI. He has written 6 books and 8 chapters. He also has operative experience, which includes over 2700 neurosurgical operations. His major research interest is epidemiological, etiological, experimental and therapeutic aspects of neurotrauma especially spinal cord injury.

# Contents

# Preface

The purpose of this book is to review all types of pituitary adenoma and describe the symptoms, epidemiology, diagnosis, management, outcome and complications of them.

Pituitary adenomas are typically benign, slow-growing tumors that arise from cells in the pituitary gland. The pituitary gland lies below the optic system, primarily the optic chiasm, and below the optic nerves and optic tracts. Thus, pituitary adenomas, the most common tumors of the hypophysis, can compress optic system and some of the main symptoms and signs in patients are visual. Therefore, measurement of visual acuity, visual fields, ophthalmoscopy and the use of Optical Coherence Tomography has a significant role in diagnosis and periodic evaluation of the patient.

Pituitary adenomas are classified based on hormone secretory products. But non-functioning adenomas are endocrine-inactive tumors. Because of physiologic effects of excess hormones, the functioning tumors present earlier than non-functioning adenomas. On the other hand, the mass effect from large pituitary adenomas may lead to the pressure symptoms, such as headaches, visual field defects, cranial nerve deficits, hypopituitarism, pituitary apoplexy or stalk effect.

The molecular mechanisms underlying the development and progression of pituitary adenoma have not yet been clearly defined. However, immunohistochemistry and ultrastructural analysis developed new insights into the pathogenesis of these tumors. The finding of specific serum markers in patients with pituitary adenoma will help physicians in the accurate diagnosis and specific treatment of patients in the future.

Diagnostic MRI of the sellar region constitutes one of the most challenging subjects in neurooncology. T1- and T2-weighted MRI in coronal and sagittal planes with and without paramagnetic contrast medium is the method of choice for imaging of the pituitary gland and the perisellar area.

During the past two decades, a number of new procedures for radiation dose delivery and fractionation have become extensively accessible. The most important progress has been in the use of stereotactic procedures to make radiotherapy targeting relatively simple and very precise. This has permitted the application of single fraction high-dose irradiation entitled stereotactic radiosurgery for brain tumors which can be given as an adjuvant or as a specific treatment modality for pituitary adenomas in patients who have had recurrence after microsurgery, or if complete tumor removal has not been possible.

Finally, visual testing, endocrine evaluation and MRI are three main tools in the pre and post treatment assessment of patients with pituitary adenoma. Considering all modalities of treatment (medical, surgical, or radiotherapy) selected for management of patients, visual assessment together with endocrine and imaging is essential in short and long term evaluation of tumors of the hypophysis.

I want to thank Ms Maja Bozicevic for helping me trough the process, InTech for giving me opportunity to work as an Editor and Prof. Ed Laws for his support.

**Vafa Rahimi-Movaghar, MD**
Associate professor of Neurosurgery
Vice-Chairman of Sina Trauma and Surgery Research Center, Department of Neurosurgery, Shariati Hospital, Tehran University of Medical Sciences, Tehran, Iran
Research Centre for Neural Repair, University of Tehran, Tehran, Iran

1

# Pituitary Adenomas and Ophthalmology

Santiago Ortiz-Perez and Bernardo Sanchez-Dalmau
*Hospital Clinic, University of de Barcelona, Ophthalmology department*
*Spain*

## 1. Introduction

Pituitary gland, also called hypophysis, is a neuroendocrine organ placed in the "sella turcica" in the skull base. This gland consists of 2 main areas, the anterior and medial part constitute the adenohypophysis, the posterior part is called neurohypophysis. Pituitary gland is in charge of the internal constancy, homeostasis and reproductive function; this is why pituitary abnormalities cause a wide spectrum of signs and symptoms.

Pituitary adenomas are a common pathology; they represent about 10% of all intracranial tumours and between 50-80% of pituitary tumours. Necropsy and imaging studies estimate an incident of 20-25% of pituitary adenomas in general population; however, only about 1/3 of them are clinically evident (Asa & Ezzat, 2009). The majority of these tumours have monoclonal origin (mutation of a single gonadotropic cell), but there are still some discrepancies about the pathogenesis of these neoplasms. The most common mutations seem in other human neoplasms are not frequent in pituitary adenomas, and only a minimum proportion of them are associated to other genetic disorders, such as MEN1 syndrome (multiple endocrine neoplasms type 1) or the Carney complex, due to mutations of the genes MEN1 and PRKAR1A (protein kinase A regulatory subunit 1A) respectively (Beckers & Daly, 2007). Hormones and growth factors involve in normal pituitary function can be also related to the growth of these tumours, although evident connection with the pathogenesis has not been demonstrated.

Symptoms related to pituitary tumours are secondary to several factors. On the one hand, many of them are *non-secreting tumours*, they can be asymptomatic or cause compression symptoms if they are big enough; on the other hand, other are *secreting tumours* and they can cause clinical syndromes derivate from the hormone activity in different target organs. Hormones secreting by these tumours are the same that the physiologic hypophysis produces. According to frequency, the most frequent tumours are prolactin (PRL)-secreting pituitary adenomas, non secreting pituitary adenomas are in second position, growth hormone (GH)-secreting tumours in third, adrenocorticotropic hormone (ACTH)-secreting tumours in fourth, and the rarest are thyroid stimulating hormone (TSH)-secreting adenomas. There are also tumour secreting different combinations of hormones, mainly GH and PRL (Table 1). In cases of fast growing or big tumours affecting surrounding structures, chiasmatic or cavernous sinus syndrome can be seen.

Two types of adenomas can be described depending on the size of the tumour, macroadenomas with more than 1 centimeter and microadenomas measuring less than 1 cm in size (figure 1). A low percentage of tumours have a malign behaviour producing metastases, central nervous system invasion and even death; nevertheless, this is very uncommon and the majority of the problems related to these tumours are due to the morbidity that they produce.

| **Cell type** | **Hormones** | **Hormone function** | **Tumour incidence** | **Clinical syndromes** |
|---|---|---|---|---|
| Adrenocorticotropic | ACTH and other peptides | Adrenal cortex; glucocorticoid metabolism | 10 – 15% | Cushing syndrome<br>Nelson syndrome |
| Somatotropic | GH | IGF-1 production. Muscle and bone growth | 10 – 15% | Acromegaly<br>Gigantism |
| Lactotropic | PRL | Lactation | 35% | Amenorrhea<br>Galactorrhea<br>Sexual dysfunction |
| Mammo-somatotropic | GH , PRL | See above | 5% | Acromegaly<br>Gigantism with hyper-PRL |
| Thyrotropic | TSH | Thyroid metabolism | 2% | Hypo - hyperthyroidism |
| Gonadotropic | FSH, LH | Sexual development. Sexual steroids metabolism | 35% | Hypogonadism<br>Mass effect<br>Hypopituitarism |

Table 1. Pituitary cells, hormones, tumours and associated clinical syndromes (Asa & Ezzat, 2002)

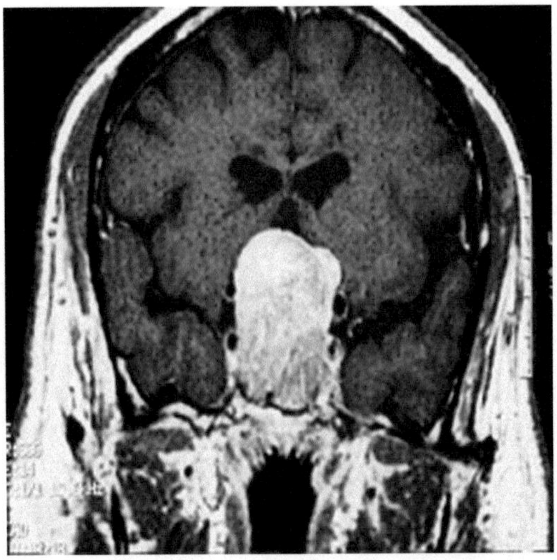

Fig. 1. Magnetic resonance imaging showing a pituitary macroadenoma.

The wide spectrum of clinical syndromes including endocrinological, cardiovascular, neurological, ophthalmological, determine the needed of a multidisciplinary management between different specialists. Early diagnosis is very important in order to establish a proper therapeutic plan and achieve the best prognosis for these patients.

In this review, a comprehensive description about the ophthalmological syndromes associated to pituitary adenomas is presented. The suspicion of these syndromes by the doctors facing patients with pituitary tumours will allow earlier diagnostic and better treatments for them. Despite the general ophthalmic examination including visual field tests, we describe the Optical Coherence Tomography (OCT) as a new tool that must be performed in all these patients.

## 2. Ophthalmic manifestations of pituitary adenomas

The most common neuro-ophthalmological syndrome associated to pituitary adenomas is due to compression of the central part of the optic chiasm; this produces the classic bitemporal hemianopia in the visual field. That was the onset manifestation in up to 80% of pituitary adenomas several years ago, but nowadays, the advantages in the hormone detection tests and neuroimaging have changed this trend, and headache and systemic clinical syndromes related to hormone production are the commonest onset manifestations. Neuro-ophthalmological manifestations are the debut syndrome in less than 10% of cases (Table 2); they are due to the anatomical relations between the gland and the optic chiasm, the optic nerves and the III, IV and VI nerves in the cavernous sinus.

| Study. No of patients Year | Amenorrhea/ Impotence(%) | Headache (%) | Visual dysfunction (%) | Optic atrophy (%) | EOM impairment |
|---|---|---|---|---|---|
| Chamblin et al (156;<1955) | -- | -- | 86 | 50 | 5 |
| Hollenhorst and younge (1000;1940-62) | 5 | 14 | 70 | 34 | 6 |
| Klauber et al (51; 1967-74) | | 45 | 69 | 47 | |
| Wray (100; 1974-76) | 21 | 24 | 31 | 19 | 4 |
| Anderson et al (200; 1976-1981) | 70 | 46 | 9 | 2 | 1 |

EOM: extraocular muscle

Table 2. Debut signs and symptoms in pituitary adenoma patients (Chhabra & Newman, 2006)

### 2.1 Anatomy of the pituitary area (Rouvière & Delmas, 1996)

Optic nerves enter the intracranial space through the *optic foramen* in the sphenoid bones, after 8-15 mm up and backwards they join together to constitute the optic chiasm. There are anatomical variations in the length of the intracranial optic nerve and the position of the optic chiasm, this is extremely important with respect to the visual deficits caused by tumours in the suprasellar region. In 75-80% of people optic chiasm is placed just above the *diaphragma sellae;* when the intracranial optic nerve is shorter than about 12 mm (about 10% of people), the optic chiasm is positioned anteriorly, or "pre-fixed", and it sits above the *tuberculum sellae,* when the intracranial optic nerve is long, over 18 mm (10-15% of people), the chiasm is positioned posteriorly to the *dorsum sellae* or "post-fixed" (Chhabra & Newman, 2006; Miller N, et al, 2008).

Fibers running from the nasal retinal nerve cells (about 53% of fibers) cross in the chiasm to join the fibers from the temporal retinal nerve cells of the opposite side. However, as they enter the chiasm, some ventral crossed fibers, primarily from the inferonasal retinal of the contralateral eye and serving the superotemporal portion of the contralateral visual field, where historically believed to loop anteriorly 1 to 2 mm into the terminal portion of the opposite optic nerve before turning posteriorly to continue through the chiasm and into the optic tract. This loop is called Willebrand's Knee (Miller N, et al, 2008; Muñoz-Negrete & Rebolleda, 2002). There is some controversy about the real anatomical existence of this structure, however Willebrand's knee clearly exists from a clinical point of view, as it is described below. In cases of chiasm compression the crossed fibers are more likely to be damaged as they support the same quantity of pressure in less space (Kosmorsky, et al, 2008). This is the reason for the bitemporal hemianopia (crossed nasal fibers compression) as the more frequent syndrome in cases of chiasm compression. Fibers leave the chiasm backwards in both sides of the hypophysis as the optic tracts; in cases of pre-fixed chiasms is more likely to see damaged of these tracts.

The pituitary gland lies between the two paired cavernous sinuses. An abnormally growing adenoma will expand in the direction of least resistance and eventually compress the cavernous sinus (figure 2). The cavernous sinus receives blood via the ophthalmic vein through the superior orbital fissure and from superficial cortical veins, and is connected to the basilar plexus of veins posteriorly. The internal carotid artery (carotid siphon), and cranial nerves III, IV, $V_1$, $V_2$ and VI all pass through this blood filled space. The cavernous sinus drains by two channels, the superior and inferior petrosal sinuses, ultimately into the internal jugular vein. These nerves, with the exception of $V_2$, pass through the cavernous sinus to enter the orbital apex through the superior orbital fissure. The maxillary nerve, division $V_2$ of the trigeminal nerve travels through the lower portion of the sinus and exits via the foramen rotundum (Miller N, et al, 2008; Frank, et al, 2006).

### 2.2 Clinical syndromes

There are different syndromes that can be seen in cases of pituitary adenomas:

#### 2.2.1 Anterior chiasmal syndrome

This is more common in post-fixed chiasms. The compression in the anterior angle of the optic chiasm affect the *Willbrandt's knee* fibers and produces temporal and superior visual field defects affecting one or both eyes. In cases of non-centred tumours the anterior junction syndrome of Traquair (junctional scotoma) can be observed, characterized by advanced visual field loss affecting the visual field centre in one eye and (possibly subtle) defects respecting the vertical midline in the fellow eye (Muñoz-Negrete & Rebolleda, 2002).

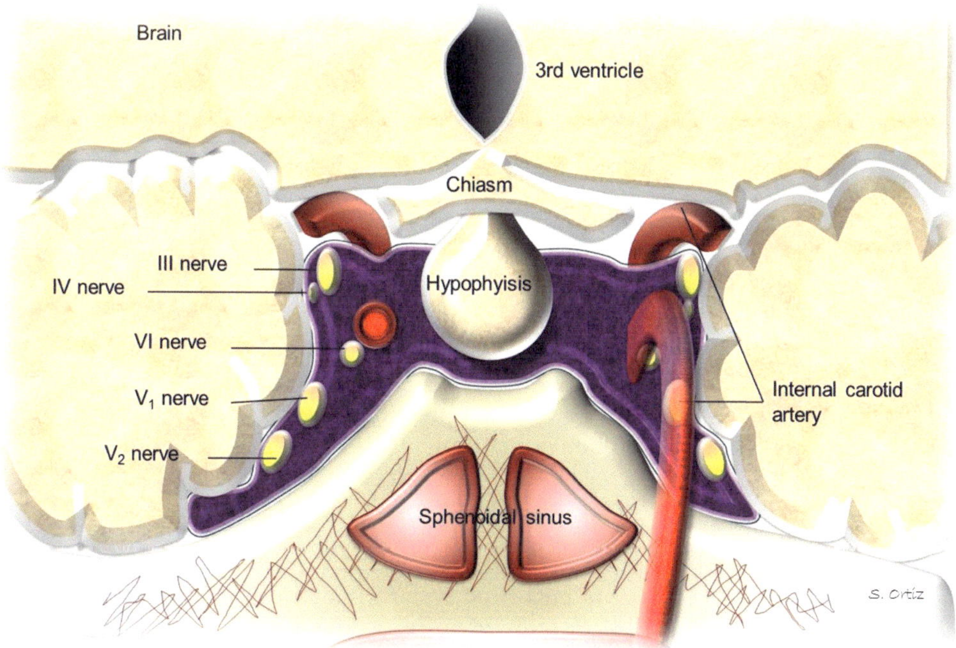


Fig. 2. Anatomy of the cavernous sinus and surrounding structures. Relation between the pituitary gland and the chiasm, cranial nerves and internal carotid arteries.

### 2.2.2 Central chiasmal syndrome

This is the most frequent syndrome; the damage involving mainly the crossed fibers produces bitemporal hemianopia with possible central visual field affectation (figure 3). This syndrome is seen in lesions that damage the body of the optic chiasm.

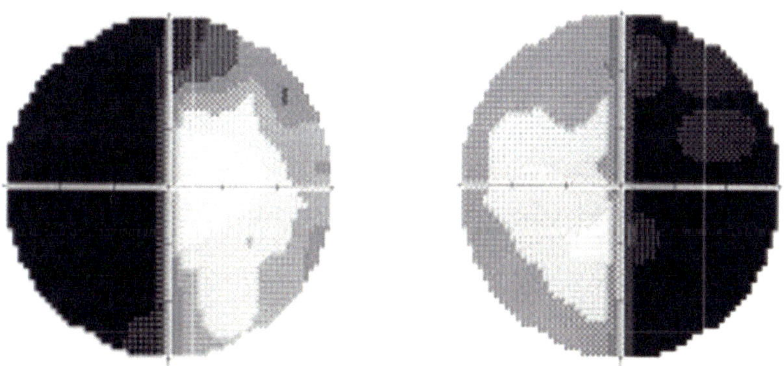

Fig. 3. Visual field showing a bitemporal hemianopia.

### 2.2.3 Inferior chiasmal syndrome

If the compression affects predominantly the inferior part of the chiasm the visual field defects are temporal and superior.

### 2.2.4 Superior chiasmal syndrome

Compression of the superior part of the chiasm is not a frequent condition in cases of pituitary adenomas; it is more likely to see this clinical picture in other tumours arising from the base of the brain, mainly the craniopharyngioma. In these cases the visual field defects are temporal and inferior.

### 2.2.5 Posterior chiasmal syndrome

More frequent in pre-fixed chiasms. It produces characteristic bitemporal hemianopic scotomas in the visual field.

### 2.2.6 Lateral chiasmal syndrome

This syndrome can be observed in tumours compressions or carotid pathology that pushes the chiasm laterally. Contralateral homonymus quadrantanopic or hemianopic defects can be assessed; much less frequent is the binasal hemianopia in these cases.

### 2.2.7 Optic tract compression

This is also more frequent in cases of post-fixed chiasms. Contralateral homonymus defects can be observed. Optic tract damage is more frequent in other neurological conditions, such as vascular processes, demyelinating diseases or trauma. Another pupillary phenomenon that is sometimes associated with lesions of the optic tract that produce a complete or nearly complete homonymus hemianopia is pupillary hemiakinesia (hemianopic pupillary reaction or Wernicke's pupil) (Miller N, et al, 2008).

### 2.2.8 Neuro-ophthalmological signs and symptoms associated with the chiasmal syndrome

The presence of visual field defect can associate different manifestations, such as the *hemifield slide phenomenon* that produces fluctuating diplopia with no oculomotor impairment due to anomalous retinal correspondence. It is also common a *disturbance of depth perception*. These two phenomenons are associated to bitemporal hemianopia (Chhabra & Newman, 2006; Miller N, et al, 2008).

### 2.2.9 Ocular motility disorders

Patients with pituitary pathology can refer diplopia related to the mentioned hemifield slide phenomenon, or due to cranial nerves damage in the cavernous sinus; the most frequently affected is the third nerve leading to an eyelid ptosis, pupillary dilation, and ocular motility disorders (figure 4). The rarest of those syndromes is the VI nerve palsy.

### 2.2.10 Nystagmus

In cases of tumours of the diencephalon and chiasmal regions the rare phenomenon of the "see-saw" nystagmus may occur. This condition is characterized by synchronous alternating elevation and incyclotorsion of one eye and depression and excyclotorsion of the opposite eye. The pathogenesis of this phenomenon is not well understood but it is thought to be related to perception impairment connected with hemianopia (Chhabra & Newman, 2006)

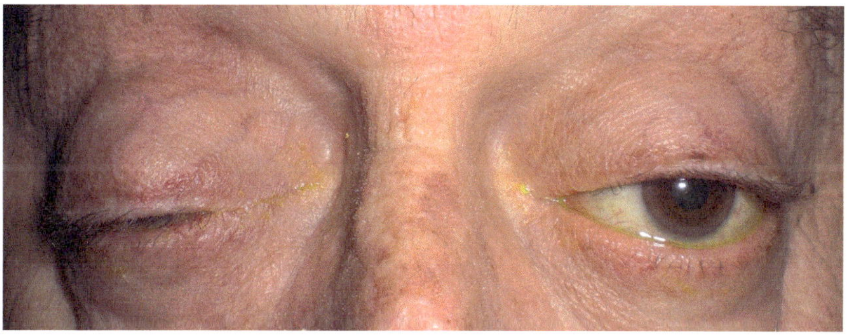

Fig. 4. Patient affected by a III nerve palsy. Observe the eyelid ptosis due to affectation of the levator muscle. These patients also have pupillary dilation and extraocular movements impairment

or damage to the interstitial nucleus of Cajal or adjacent structures of the tumour (Miller, et al, 2008). In cases of big tumours compressing the brainstem is also possible, although exceptional, the presence of nystagmus.

### 2.2.11 Colour vision impairment

This can be observed as a sign of visual pathway damage in different conditions, including cases of pituitary adenomas.

### 2.2.12 Photophobia

Some authors suggest that persistent photophobia of unknown aetiology should arise the suspicion of pituitary pathology (Kawasaki & Purvin, 2002).

### 2.2.13 Pituitary apoplexy

Defined as a sudden neurologic impairment, usually due to a vascular process. It is characterized by a sudden onset of headache, visual symptoms, altered mental status, and hormonal dysfunction due to acute hemorrhage or infarction of a pituitary gland. An existing pituitary adenoma is usually present. The incidence of this phenomenon has been described up to 10% in some series (Wakai, 1981). The visual symptoms may include both visual acuity impairment and visual field impairment from involvement of the optic nerve or chiasm and ocular motility dysfunction from involvement of the cranial nerves traversing the cavernous sinus (more frequent III nerve). Other less common symptoms are related to possible brainstem damage, such as light-near dissociation or convergence retraction nystagmus.

### 2.2.14 Funduscopy

Most of the cases show normal optic discs in fundus examination. If altered, it can be a diffuse atrophy, or more typically the "band" or "bow-tie" atrophy that occupies a more or less horizontal band across the disc with relative sparing of the superior and inferior portions where the majority of spared temporal fibers enter (figure 5). Some cases can develop papilledema, this is more frequently associated with suprachiasmal tumours that can invade and compress the 3rd ventricle, ultimately obstructing the flow of cerebrospinal fluid.

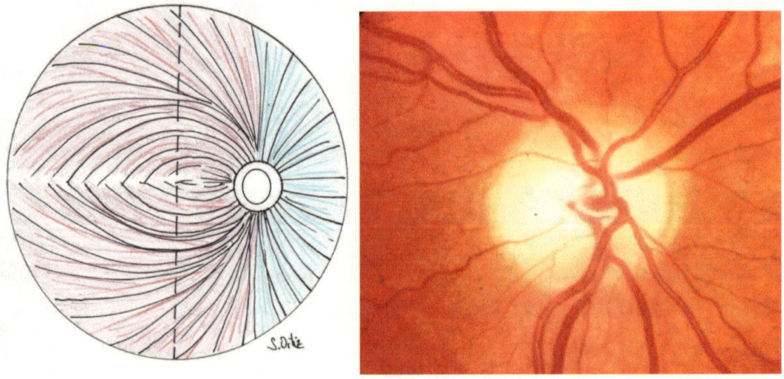

Fig. 5. Schematic representation of retinal nerve fibers (A). Optic disc of a patient with a pituitary adenoma showing atrophy of the nasal and temporal areas ("band" atrophy) and relative spare of the superior and inferior areas of the disc (B).

### 2.2.15 Other neuro-ophthalmological manifestations

Apart from the syndromes derivated from the tumour itself, the treatments used in these patients can produce neuro-ophthalmological side-effects:

- Toxic dopaminergic psychosis caused by *Bromocriptine*. Treatment with this drug can also produce a quick tumour regression leading to an *empty sella syndrome* due to a herniation of the chiasm.
- The surgical treatment most frequently performed today for these patients is the endoscopic trans-sphenoidal surgery. This technique can be also responsible for some ophthalmological side effects, mainly for damaging the optic nerves or the chiasm; nevertheless, the increasingly improvement in the equipment and surgical techniques allows treatments with much less complications (Cappabianca, et al, 2002).
- Post-radiotherapy optic neuropathy. This is a minor problem nowadays because radiotherapy is an unusual treatment for these tumours, and also because of the improvement in the techniques using fractioned radiotherapy and protecting important structures such as the optic discs (Van den Bergh, et al, 2007).

## 3. Visual recovery prediction factors

During the last years different specialists involve in the management of pituitary adenomas have tried to establish prognostic factors of visual recovery after the treatment of these patients. To date there are several well recognize prognostic factors, such as the age of patients (the older the worse prognostic), the duration of the symptoms before the surgery, the size of the tumour (better prognostic in microadenomas) and the presence of pituitary apoplexy, which is a bad prognostic factor. From the ophthalmology point of view, several factors such as visual acuities less than 20/100 or a pale optic disc have been reported to determine a worse prognostic (Chhabra & Newman, 2006).

Although some cases show a severe visual impairment, it is not unusual to observe important early recoveries (1st week), intermediate recoveries (1-4 months) or even late recoveries in some patients (up to 36 months after surgery) (Kerrison, et al, 2000). This indicates that there must be other factors that determine different degrees of axonal affectation in different patients. One of the main current research lines in this field is actually seeking the diagnostic tools that allow us to predict the degree of axonal loss, and so the possibility of visual function recovery after the treatment.

During the last years, OCT has been used to establish and quantifying the axonal loss in several neurological disorders. OCT is a non-invasive tool that allows the retina to be directly approached as an appendix of the central nervous system. We can measure peripapillary retinal nerve fiber layer (RNFL) thickness, a parameter which has been found to be reproducible and useful for the diagnosis, prognosis and follow-up of optic nerve axonal damage in several neurological diseases, including pituitary adenomas (Moura, et al, 2007; Parisi, 2003; Sergott, et al, 2007; Kallenbach & Frederiksen, 2007; Toledo, et al, 2008; Noval, et al, 2006; Vessani, et al, 2009). (figure 6). OCT can be useful predicting

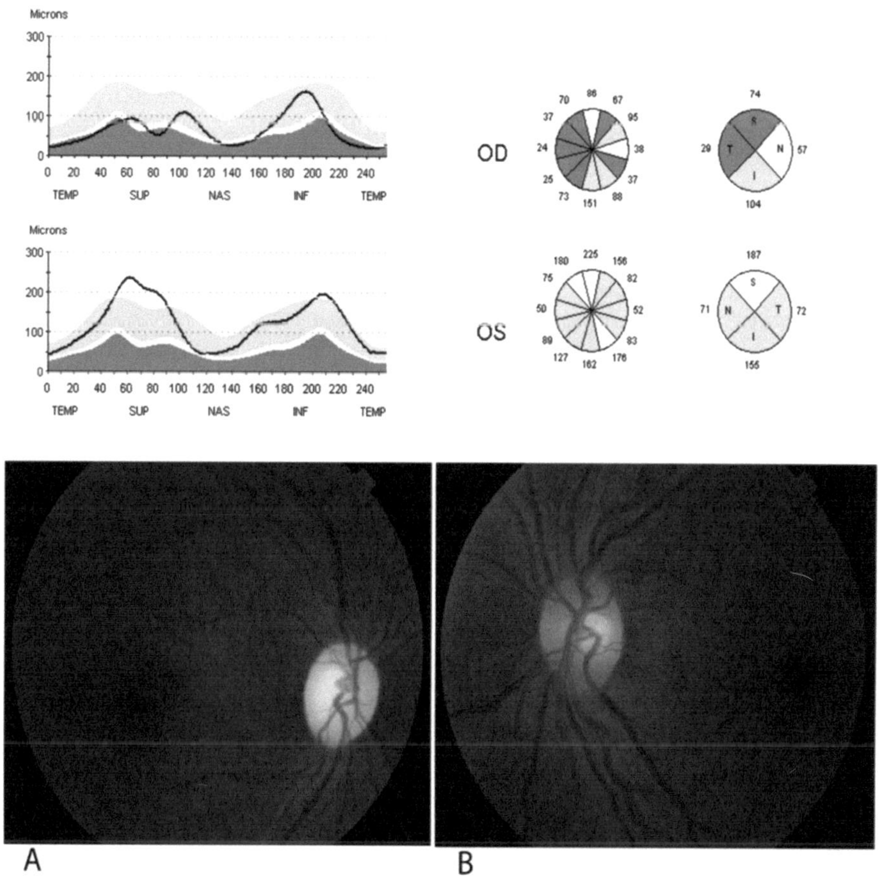


Fig. 6. Optical Coherence Tomography. Observe the retinal nerve fiber layer (RNFL) measurement in microns. A diagram is included to analyze the different sectors of the optic disc and peripapillar area. This example shows thinning of the RNFL affecting the right eye (OD) predominantly in the superior and temporal quadrants, the left eye (OS) shows normal results. The bottom of the image shows funduscopy of both eyes and demonstrates the optic disc atrophy of the right eye (A) while the left eye is normal (B).

the visual function recovery in patients with pituitary adenomas by measuring the axonal damage in the retina during the evolution of the disease (Ortiz-Perez, et al, 2009; Jacob, et al, 2008).

## 4. Conclusions

Pituitary adenomas are a frequent pathology with a wide spectrum of clinical features. These tumours should be managed between different specialists including general practitioners, endocrinologists, neurologists, neurosurgeons and ophthalmologists. Neuro-ophthalmological manifestations of pituitary adenomas are frequent and varied. They represent sometimes the onset symptoms in these patients. Many of the syndromes described above have an important diagnostic value due to their localizing information. Physicians must be aware about these syndromes in order to refer patients for ophthalmological assessments and establish an early diagnosis.

OCT is a new device used daily in ophthalmology clinics to study the retina and optic disc. This tool gives unique and new information about the axonal loss in patients with neurological disorders, including pituitary adenomas. OCT is easily performed, it has no side effects or contraindications, so it must be included in the routine examination of patients with hypophysis tumours.

## 5. References

Asa, SL. & Ezzat, S. (2009). The pathogenesis of pituitary tumors. *Annu Rev Pathol,* Vol. 4 (2009), pp. (97-126)

Beckers, A. & Daly, AF. (2007). The clinical, pathological, and genetic features of familial isolated pituitary adenomas. *Eur J Endocrinol,* Vol. 157, 4, (Oct 2007), pp. (371-82).

Cappabianca, P., Cavallo, LM., Colao, AM. & de Divitiis, E. (2002). Surgical complications associated with the endoscopic endonasal transsphenoidal approach for pituitary adenomas. *J Neurosurg*. Vol. 97, 2, (Aug 2002), pp. (293-298).

Chhabra, VS. & Newman, NJ. (2006). The neuro-ophthalmology of pituitary tumors. *Compr Ophthalmol Update,* Vol. 7, 5, (Oct 2006), pp. (225-240).

Frank, G., Pasquini, E., Farneti, G., Mazzatenta, D., Sciarretta, V., Grasso, V. & Faustini, M. (2006). The endoscopic versus the traditional approach in pituitary surgery. *Neuroendocrinology*. Vol. 83, 3-4, (2006), pp. (240-248).

Jacob, M., Joaunneau, E. & Raverot, G. (2008). Value of optical coherence tomography (OCT) in predicting visual outcome after treatment of pituitary adenoma. In: *North American Neuro-Ophthalmology Society (NANOS) congress*. Orlando, EEUU, March 2008.

Kallenbach, K. & Frederiksen, J. (2007). Optical coherence tomography in optic neuritis and multiple sclerosis: a review. *Eur J Neurol*. Vol. 14, 8, (Aug 2007), pp. (841-849).

Kawasaki, A. & Purvin, VA. (2002). Photophobia as the presenting visual symptom of chiasmal compression. *J Neuroophthalmol*. Vol. 22, 1, (Mar 2002), pp. (3-8).

Kerrison, JB., Lynn, MJ., Baer, CA., Newman, SA., Biousse, V. & Newman, NJ. (2000). Stages of improvement in visual fields after pituitary tumors resection. *Am J Ophthalmol.* Vol. 130, 6, (Dec 2000), pp. (813-820).

Kosmorsky, GS., Dupps, WJ Jr. & Drake, RL. (2008). Nonuniform pressure generation in the optic chiasm may explain bitemporal hemianopsia. *Ophthalmology.* Vol. 115, 3, (Mar 2008), pp. (560-565).

Miller, NR., Newman, NJ., Biousse, V. & Kerrison, JB. *Walsh and Hoyt's Clinical Neuro-Ophthalmology: the essentials* (2nd ed), Lippincott Williams & Wilkins, ISBN-13: 978-0-7817-6379-0, Philadelphia.

Moura, FC., Medeiros, FA. & Monteiro, ML. (2007). Evaluation of macular thickness measurements for detection of band atrophy of the optic nerve using optical coherente tomography. *Ophthalmology.* Vol. 114, 1, (Jan 2007), pp. (175-181).

Muñoz-Negrete, FJ. & Rebolleda, G. (2002). Automated perimetry and neuro-ophthalmology. Topographic correlation. *Arch Soc Esp Oftalmol,* Vol. 77, 8, (Aug 2002), pp. (413-428).

Noval, S., Contreras, I., Rebolleda, G. & Muñoz-Negrete, FJ. (2006). Optical coherence tomography versus automated perimetry for follow-up of optic neuritis. *Acta Ophthalmol Scand.* Vol. 84, 6, (Dec 2008), pp. (790-794).

Ortiz-Pérez, S., Sánchez-Dalmau, BF., Molina-Fernández, JJ. & Adán-Civera, A. (2009). Neuro-ophthalmological manifestations of pituitary adenomas. The usefulness of optical coherence tomography. *Rev Neurol.* Vol. 48, 2, (Jan 2009), pp. (85-90).

Parisi, V. Correlation between morphological and functional retinal impairment in patients affected by ocular hypertension, glaucoma, demyelinating optic neuritis and Alzheimer's disease. *Semin Ophthalmol.* Vol. 18, 2, (Jun 2003), pp. (50-57).

Rouvière, H. & Delmas, A. (1996). *Anatomía Humana. Descriptiva, topográfica y funcional* (9th ed), Masson, ISBN 84-458-0506-1, Barcelona.

Sergott, RC., Frohman, E., Glanzman, R. & Al-Sabbagh, A. (2007). The role of optical coherence tomography in multiple sclerosis: expert panel consensus. *J Neurol Sci.* Vol. 263, 1-2, (Dec 2007), pp. (3-14).

Toledo, J., Sepulcre, J., Salinas-Alaman, A. Garcia-Layana, A,. Murie-Fernandez, M,. Bejarano, B. & Villoslada, P. (2008). Retinal nerve fiber layer atrophy is associated with physical and cognitive disability in multiple sclerosis. *Mult Scler.* Vol. 14, 7, (Aug 2008), pp. (906-912).

Van den Bergh, AC., Van den Berg, G., Schoorl, MA., Sluiter, WJ., Van der Vliet, AM., Hoving, EW., Szabó, BG, Langendijk, JA,. Wolffenbuttel, BH. & Dullart, RP. (2007). Immediate postoperative radiotherapy in residual nonfunctioning pituitary adenoma: beneficial effect on local control without additional negative impact on pituitary function and life expectancy. *Int J Radiat Oncol Biol Phys.* Vol. 67, 3, (Mar 2007), pp. (863-869).

Vessani, RM., Moritz, R., Batis, L., Zagui, RB., Bernardoni, S. & Susanna, R. (2009). Comparison of quantitative imaging devices and subjective optic nerve head assessment by general ophthalmologists to differentiate normal from glaucomatous eyes. *J Glaucoma.* Vol. 18, 3, (Mar 2009), pp. (253-261).

Wakai, S., Fukushima, T., Teramoto, A. & Sano, K. (1981). Pituitary apoplexy: its incidence and clinical significance. *J Neurosurg*. Vol. 55, 2, (Aug 1981), pp. (187-193).

2

# Diagnostic Imaging of the Pituitary and Parasellar Region

Joanna Bladowska and Marek Sąsiadek
*Department of General Radiology, Interventional Radiology and Neuroradiology*
*Wroclaw Medical University*
*Poland*

## 1. Introduction

Pituitary (*hypophysis*), the secreting gland located in the sella turcica, has fascinated the scientists since ages. In 1543 the Belgian scientist Andreas Vesalius described the anatomy of pituitary gland for the first time. He believed that pituitary produces mucus, which is secreted from the brain into the nasal cavity. This is why pituitary was called the mucous gland (*glandula pituitaria; pituita = mucus*). Pituitary gland, also called as „master gland" plays the special role in the body. There are plenty of pathological changes with different clinical and radiological appearances of lesions located in sellar and parasellar region. The knowledge of pituitary anatomy and function, as well as of the characteristic changes in size and shape of the pituitary throughout the life and special physiologic conditions, is mandatory for the correct diagnosis and therefore these factors have to be taken into account before assessing pituitary abnormalities.

## 2. Imaging of pituitary gland

Introduction of imaging modalities, especially magnetic resonance (MR), and of modern methods of neurosurgery and pharmacotherapy revolutionised diagnosis and therapy of pituitary tumours. Currently, MR is the method of choice for imaging of the pituitary gland and the parasellar area. Advanced MR techniques - MR diffusion, MR spectroscopy and MR perfusion - have been increasingly applied (Boxerman et al., 2010; Chernov et al., 2009).

MR imaging protocol of pituitary and sellar region including postoperative studies should consist of unenhanced T1 and T2-weighted images in coronal and sagittal planes (slice thickness 3mm, field of view FOV=16x16). Paramagnetic contrast medium is administrated intravenously at the standard dose of 0.1 ml/kg BM and post-contrast T1-weighted images are taken in coronal and sagittal planes (Bladowska et al., 2004, 2011).

MR examination enables visualization of many anatomic details of pituitary gland, such as: the anterior lobe (adenohypophysis), the posterior lobe (neurohypophysis), pituitary infundibulum, parasellar structures (cavernous sinuses, sphenoid sinus, suprasellar cisterns) and optic chiasm (Bladowska et al., 2004).

The normal pituitary gland shows the homogenous signal intensity, which is isointense compared to the white matter signal on T1-weighted as well as on T2-weighted images

(Fig.1a,b). After contrast administration pituitary gland presents the homogenous strong enhancement (Fig.2a,b).

The posterior lobe of the pituitary demonstrates the characteristic high signal intensity on T1- and T2-weighted images, seen just in front of the sellar dorsum and clearly differentiated from the anterior pituitary lobe. The high signal intensity of the posterior lobe is especially clearly visible on the sagittal planes (Fig. 3a,b) and it is called "posterior pituitary bright spot". This high intensity signal observed in the posterior lobe is believed to be related to intracellular droplets of lipid or lipidlike material in pituicytes (astrocytic glial cells). However, the recent studies using the sequences with fat suppression have not confirmed the presence of fat tissue within the neurohypophysis (Arslan et al., 1999).

Absence of this high intensity signal have been reported in patients with central diabetes insipidus (Fig.4a.b). It has to be stressed that some normal subjects lack this hyperintense

A B

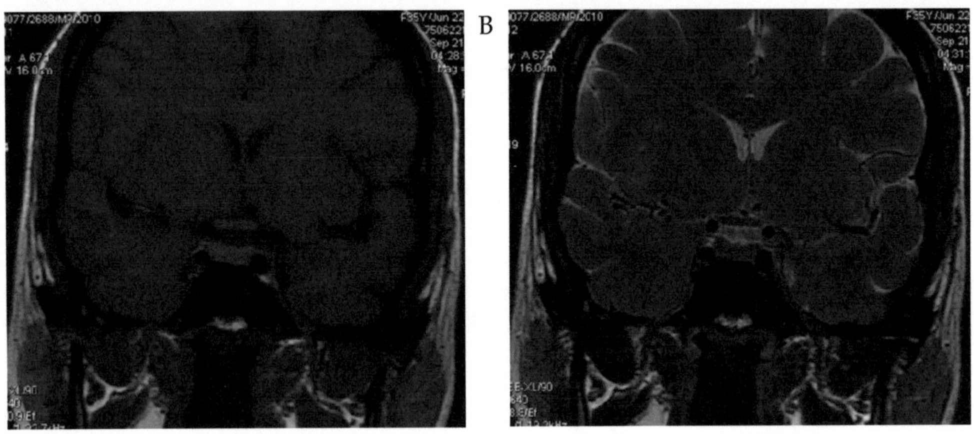

Fig. 1. MR imaging of normal pituitary gland in coronal planes before contrast administration: A. T1-weighted image. B. T2-weighted image.

A B

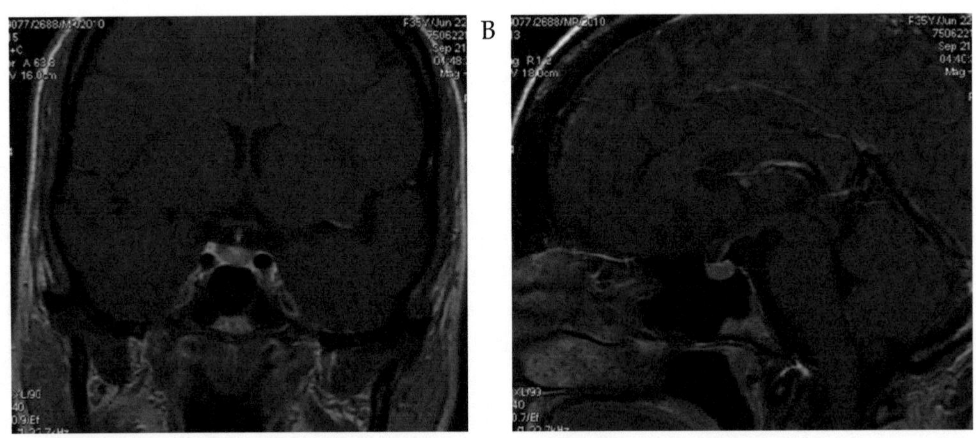

Fig. 2. MR imaging of normal pituitary gland, T1-weighted images after contrast administration: A. Coronal plane. B. Sagittal plane.

A B
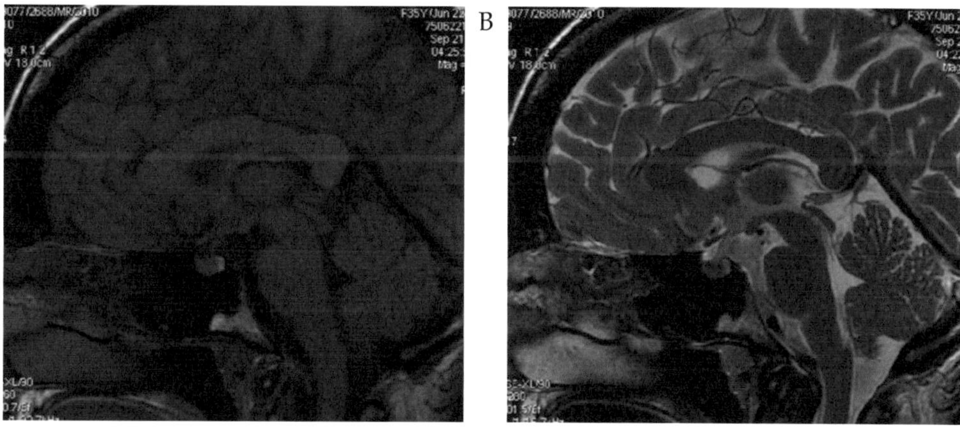

Fig. 3. MR imaging of normal pituitary gland in sagittal planes before contrast administration: A. T1-weighted image. B. T2-weighted image. The high signal intensity of the posterior lobe is clearly visible.

A B
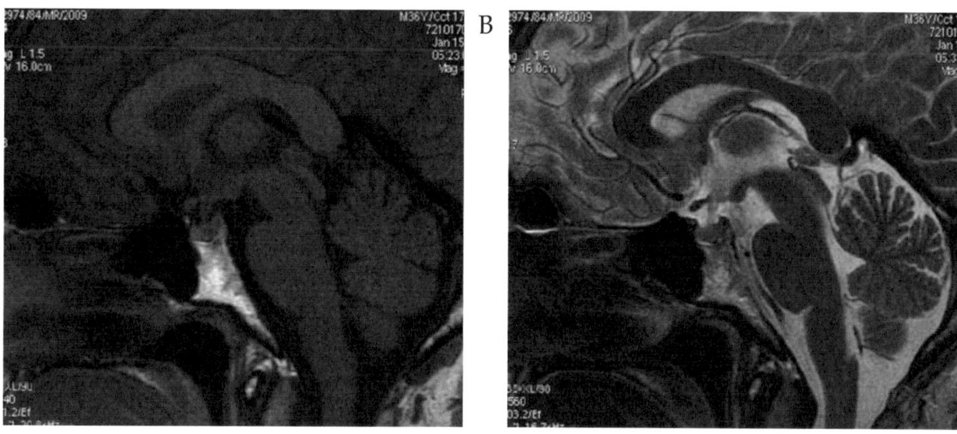

Fig. 4. MR imaging in sagittal planes before contrast administration, a 36-y.o. man with central diabetes insipidus. A. T1-weighted image. B. T2-weighted image. The high signal intensity of the posterior lobe is not visible.

signal of the posterior lobe, therefore its absence cannot be taken as an absolute sign of pituitary disease or dysfunction (Evanson, 2002).

The normal pituitary gland undergoes the characteristic changes in size and shape throughout the life, which have to be taken into account before assessing pituitary abnormalities.

In neonates, the pituitary gland is typically convex and shows a higher signal intensity compared to the brain stem on T1-weighted images (Fig.5). This appearance persists for about 2 months, after which the pituitary will present with a flat superior surface and a signal intensity similar to the signal of the pons, what is typical for the older children.

Throughout childhood, the pituitary reveals a slight but definite growth in all dimensions. The upper surface is flat or mildly concave and the height of the pituitary in the sagittal plane is about 2-6mm (Fig.6a,b), there are no differences between girls and boys.

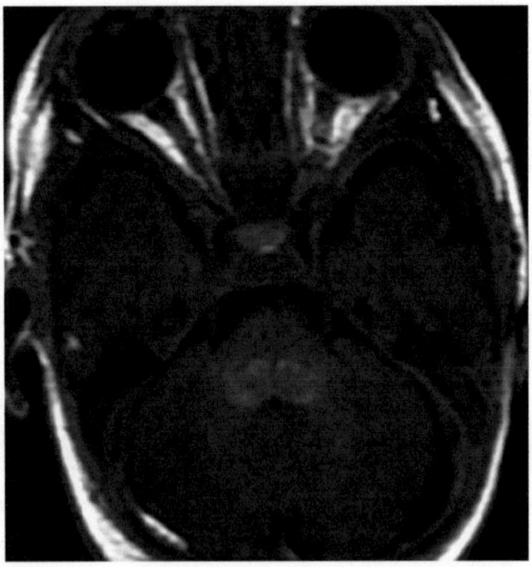

Fig. 5. MR imaging in neonate, T1-weighted image in axial plane. The pituitary gland demonstrates the characteristic high signal intensity.

A

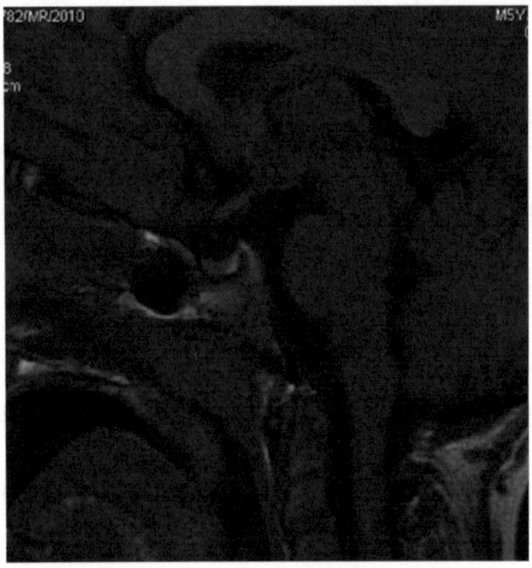

B

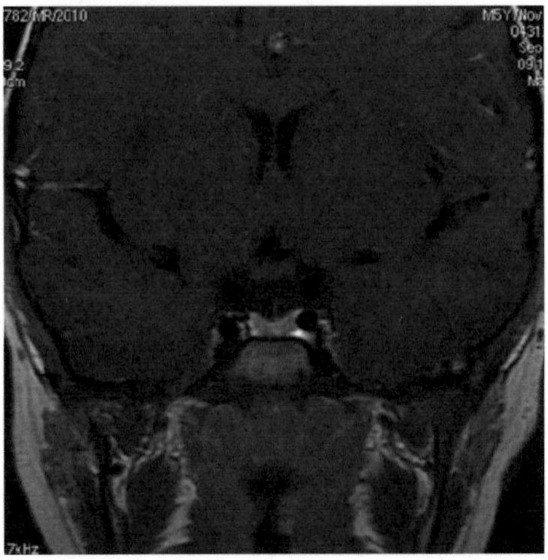

Fig. 6. MR imaging of normal pituitary gland in 5-y.o. boy, T1-weighted images.: A. Sagittal plane B. Coronal plane after contrast administration.

At puberty the pituitary gland demonstrates the huge changes in size and shape, becoming larger than at any other time of the whole life. In girls the gland can reach the height of 10mm, while in boys it may measure 7-8mm. Furthermore, in pubertal girls the gland can also project above the sella and present with a marked convexity of its superior surface (Elster, 1990, 1993).

Physiologic hypertrophy of the pituitary can be observed during pregnancy, when the gland may increase in weight by 30%-100%. By the third trimester the pituitary usually measures even 10mm of height and shows the typical convex superior surface. It has to be stressed that during pregnancy and the 1st postpartum week, the pituitary gland demonstrates the high signal intensity on T1-weighted images (Fig.7), like in the neonate period (Bladowska et al., 2004; Elster, 1991, 1993).

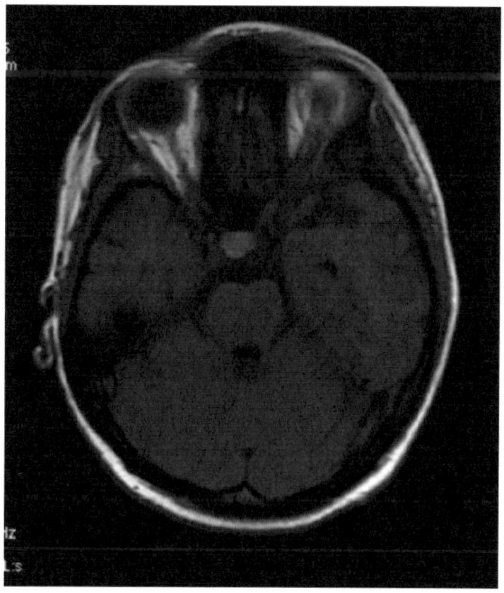

Fig. 7. MR imaging of the pituitary gland in 24-y.o. woman 5 days after delivery, T1-weighted image in axial plane. The pituitary gland demonstrated the characteristic high signal intensity.

From young adulthood until middle age, the pituitary glands of both sexes show usually stable appearance. Beyond age of 50 years, progressive involution of the gland is observed, what is probably related to the decrease in pituitary activity during menopause and andropause period. It has to be emphasized that in about 30% of this population the high signal intensity of the posterior pituitary lobe is not visible, as well as the empty sella syndrome is more commonly noted, but these changes are typical signs of normal aging process (Bladowska et al., 2004; Elster, 1993).

## 3. Imaging of pituitary adenomas

Pituitary adenomas constitute approximately 10 to 15% of all primary intracranial neoplasms and are the most common causes of pituitary function disorders and field of view deficits. Therefore, early diagnosis and therapy of patients with pituitary tumors are of high importance in clinical practice (Bladowska et al., 2010a).

Pituitary adenomas are the most common pathology encountered in the sellar region. They are usually benign and slow growing tumors, but up to 50% reveal histological evidence of capsule invasion, furthermore less than 0.2% could be malignant, causing local spread into the central nervous system. Pituitary carcinoma is exceedingly rare.

About 70% of pituitary adenomas are diagnosed in patients aged 30-50-y.o., while subjects in age below 20-y.o. constitute only 3 to 7% of all patients with pituitary tumors. Besides, pituitary adenomas are more common in women than in men (Daly et al., 2009).

Pituitary adenomas can be classified on the basis of their size: microadenomas are less than 10mm in diameter and macroadenomas are greater than 10mm. It has to be stressed that the separate term "picoadenomas" should be used for describing the tumors smaller than 3mm, because these lesions are posing special diagnostic problems – it is often impossible to visualize the picoadenomas on MR imaging (Bonneville et al., 2000, 2005).

Furthermore, clinically adenomas are classified depending upon the presence or absence of specific hormonal activity. They are divided into two groups: functioning pituitary adenomas and non-functioning adenomas. Functioning adenomas usually secrete a single hormone causing a well recognised endocrine syndrome like e.g. acromegaly (GH - growth hormone-secreting adenomas).

In MR imaging, on T1-weighted images, about 80-90% of pituitary microadenomas present with lower signal intensity compared to the normal anterior pituitary lobe – they are hypointense. The other cases of microadenomas could be isointense and therefore they will be not visible on T1-weighted images before contrast administration. Pituitary microadenomas can also reveal high signal intensity on T1-weighted images, what may be caused by hemorrhagic transformation of the adenoma and this is a frequent sign in prolactinomas (PRL - prolactine-secreting adenomas). On T2-weighted images, about 1/3 to ½ of microadenomas demonstrate high signal intensity (Fig.8), what is especially helpful in making the correct diagnosis of pituitary pathology. Increased signal intensity on T2-weighted images is noted in over 80% of microprolactinomas. The other types of pituitary microadenomas can present different signal intensity on T2- weighted images, iso or hypointense signal occurs in about 2/3 cases of GH-secreting microadenomas (Bonneville et al., 2005).

A B

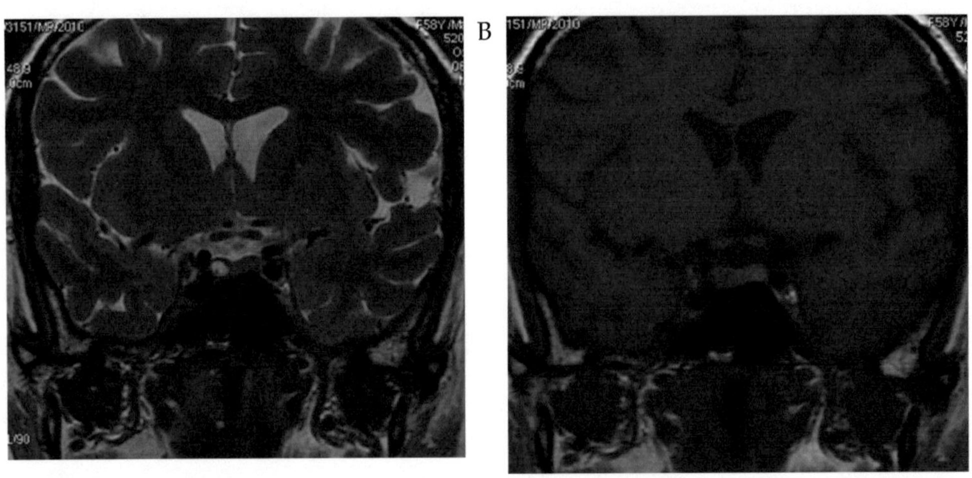

Fig. 8. MR imaging in coronal planes before contrast administration. A. T2-weighted image. B. T1-weighted image. On the right side of the pituitary gland there is a microadenoma, which shows the high signal intensity on T2- weighted image, making the correct diagnosis easy, while it is almost not visible on T1-weighted image.

On the contrast-enhanced T1-weighted images microadenomas can show typically low signal intensity compared to the intense enhancement of the unaffected pituitary gland (Fig.9) (Bladowska et al., 2004).

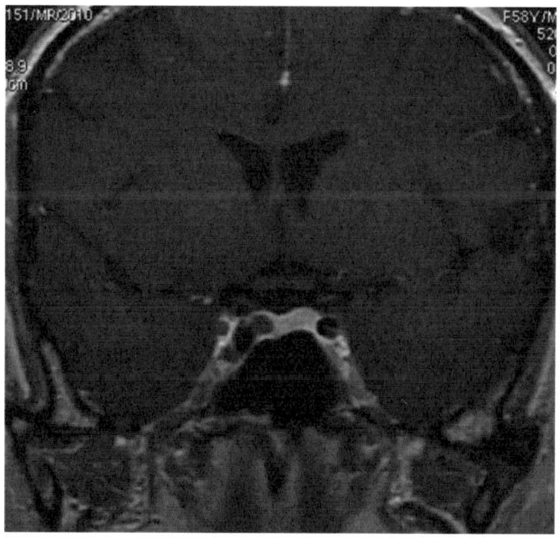

Fig. 9. T1-weighted image in coronal plane after contrast administration. The hypointense microadenoma is visible on the right side of the pituitary gland.

It has to be emphasized, as mentioned above, the contrast-enhancement images may be normal in case of the extremely small tumor (picoadenoma). When the plain MR images are not convincing, other techniques can be also used. The delayed images taken about 30-40 minutes after contrast administration may reveal late enhancement of the microadenoma itself (Bonneville et al., 2005). In our own material of pituitary adenomas we have noticed microadenomas, which show contrast-enhancement just about 10 minutes after injection of contrast (Fig.10a,b).

A

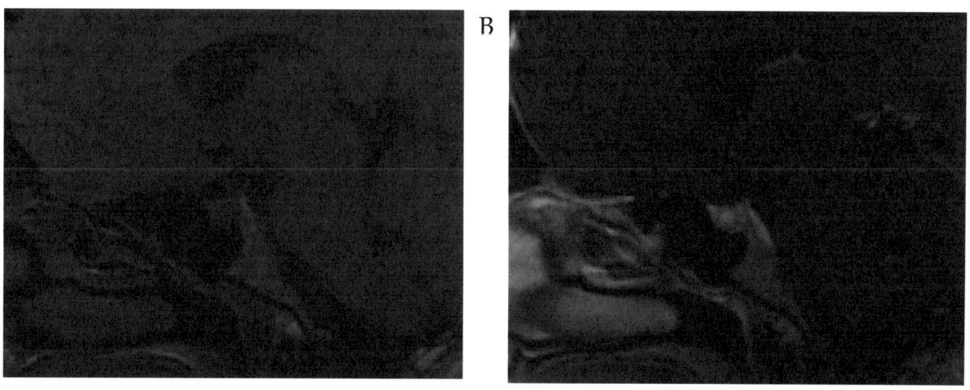


Fig. 10. T1-weighted sagittal images, before (A) and about 10 minutes after contrast administration. On the delayed image the enhancing microadenoma is clearly visible.

The ACTH-secreting microadenomas associated with Cushing's disease tend to be very small (typical feature of picoadenomas) and more often occult on MR imaging (Bonneville et al., 2005; Evanson, 2002). Dynamic imaging can be recommended in the diagnosis of ACTH-secreting microadenomas, when the clinical symptoms are highly suggesting of pituitary pathology, but the plain MR imaging is normal. Dynamic imaging can evidence a lack or a temporary delay of enhancement in the microadenoma compared to the unaffected pituitary gland. However, the delayed images taken at least about 10 minutes after contrast administration seem to be more useful in inconclusive cases.

The diagnosis of macroadenoma in MR imaging is usually simple because of the tumor size over 10mm, making the adenoma clearly visible, even in the computed tomography (CT). However, the other tumors may also be located in the sellar region and they can mimic pituitary adenomas. Therefore, the precise knowledge of the MR appearance of the macroadenomas is of high importance in the clinical practice.

Macroadenomas are usually isointense on T1-weighted images, and after contrast administration they show different enhancement patterns (Fig.11, 12). On T2-weighted images they may be often inhomogenous, with disseminated high intensity areas of cystic degeneration or necrotic regions. About 18% of macroadenomas reveal the cystic components, while about 20% show features of haemorrhage, usually clinically asymptomatic and diagnosed incidentally in MR imaging. Large pituitary adenomas are prone to develop infarction or haemorrhage, because of their tenuous blood supply.

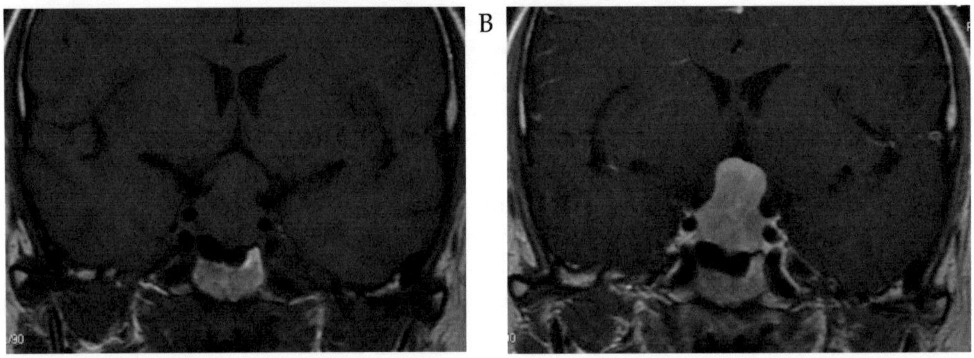

Fig. 11. T1-weighted coronal images before (A) and after contrast administration (B). The sellar-suprasellar macroadenoma shows strong contrast-enhancement. There is evidence of the optic chiasm and the third ventricle compression.

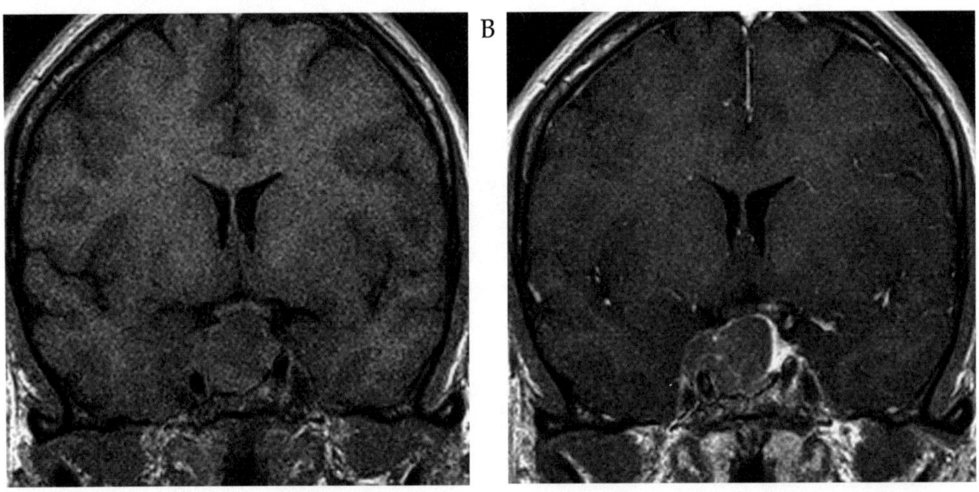

Fig. 12. T1-weighted coronal images before (A) and after contrast administration (B). The macroadenoma does not enhance after contrast injection. The compressed pituitary gland, showing the high signal intensity, is displaced to the left side of the sella. There is also the right cavernous sinus involvement.

Intratumoral hemorrhage is very often found in prolactinomas, especially after the treatment with bromocriptine. However, the hemorrhage may be revealed on MR images within adenomas in patients, who have not been treated (Bonneville et al., 2005). The hemorrhage shows the characteristic high intensity signal on T1-weighted images (Fig.13). A "fluid-fluid level" can be seen within the hemorrhage, and this feature is typical and more common in adenomas compared to other tumors, such as craniopharyngiomas.

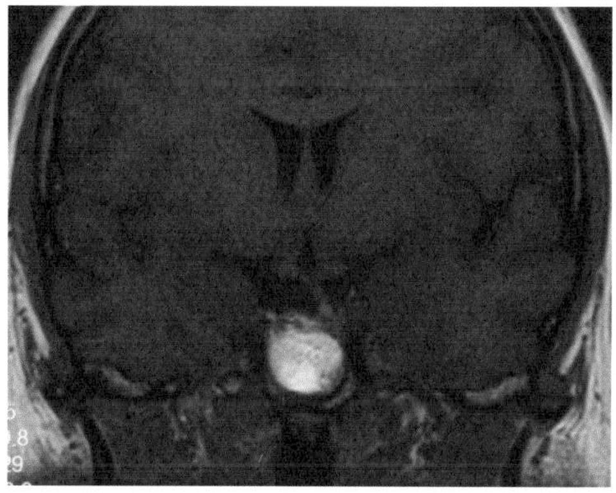

Fig. 13. T1-weighted coronal unenhanced image. The high intensity area of hemorrhage within prolactine-secreting macroadenoma is visible.

Macroadenomas are intrasellar masses usually with extrasellar extension. They may grow upwards causing the optic chiasm compression and indent the floor of the third ventricle. These tumors can also extend downward into the sphenoid sinus, back into the dorsum sellae or laterally into the cavernous sinus. Involvement of the cavernous sinus can modify the prognosis, therefore the correct diagnosis is of high clinical importance, although it may remain difficult to differentiate compression and involvement. The complete encasement of the intracavernous part of the internal carotid artery (ICA) by the adenoma is the best sign of involvement of the cavernous sinus (Fig.14) (Bladowska et al., 2004).

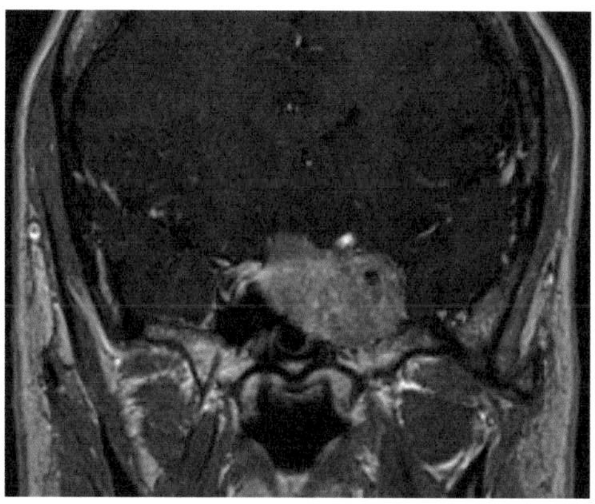

Fig. 14. T1-weighted coronal contrast-enhanced image. The complete encasement of the intracavernous part of the left internal carotid artery by the adenoma is visible.

## 4. Imaging of other pituitary tumors and parasellar lesions

The most common pituitary tumors are adenomas, the other tumors constitute approximately 5 to 10% of all sellar and parasellar lesions. The precise knowledge of the MR appearance of these lesions is of high importance in clinical practice, because they can mimic pituitary adenomas. In this subsection we describe the characteristic imaging features of these tumors.

### 4.1 Craniopharyngiomas

Craniopharyngiomas are the most common suprasellar lesions. They account for approximately 3% of all intracranial neoplasms and are slow-growing, benign tumors, which arise from squamous epithelial cell rests of Rathke's pouch. These tumors are frequent in children and young adults, but they also can be found in older adults. Craniopharyngiomas may be divided into two histological types: adamantinomatous and squamous-papillary (Doerfler & Richter, 2008).

In MR imaging the signal intensity of craniopharyngioma varies with cyst contents. High T1 signal is the results of high protein content (Fig.15). The classic adamantinomatous type usually consists of hyperintense cysts and heterogeneous nodules. The less common papillary type is presented with isointense solid component. On T2-weighted images cysts are predominantly hyperintense, while the solid components show heterogeneous signal. After contrast administration the solid portions enhance heterogeneously, as well as cysts walls reveal strong enhancement (Bladowska et al. 2004; Doerfler & Richter, 2008).

A B

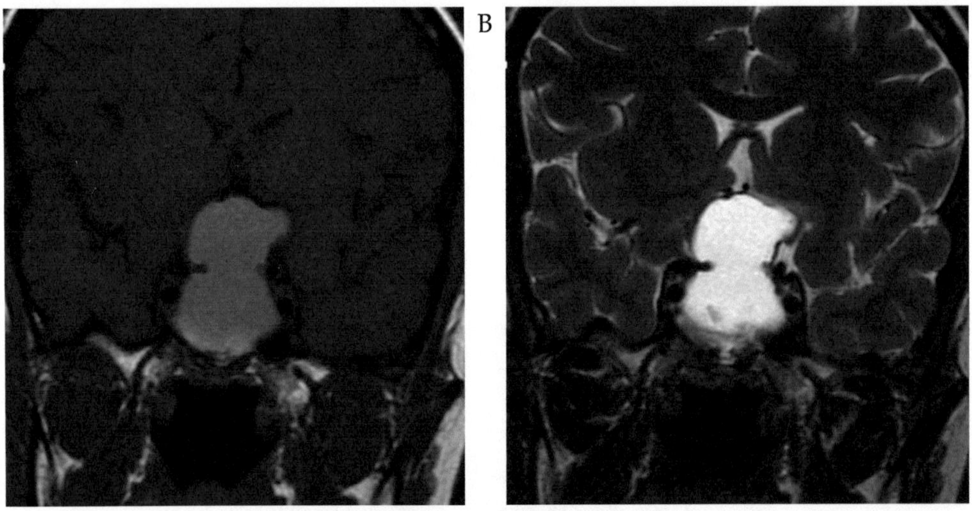

Fig. 15. MR imaging in coronal planes before contrast administration. A. T1-weighted image. B. T2-weighted image. The sellar-suprasellar craniopharyngioma presents with high signal intensity on both T1- and T2-weighted images.

### 4.2 Rathke's Cleft Cyst

Rathke's cleft cysts account for approximately 1.5% of all sellar and parasellar lesions. They, like craniopharyngiomas, are also derived from the Rathke's pouch, but are usually smaller and almost always located intrasellar, between the anterior and posterior pituitary lobe.

Furthermore, they present with different histological structure compared to craniopharyngiomas - Rathke's cysts are lined by a single layer of epithelium, while craniopharyngiomas have thick walls composed of squamous or basal cells (Bladowska et al. 2004; Doerfler & Richter, 2008).

Rathke's cleft cysts are relatively common incidental findings, usually remaining asymptomatic.

In MR imaging Rathke's cleft cysts display variable signal intensity. Cysts containing serous fluid are typically hypointense on T1-weighted images and hyperintense on T2-weighted images (Fig.16), while mucoid cyst reveal high signal intensity on T1-weighted images and often characteristic very low signal on T2-weighted images (Fig.17). After contrast administration they usually do not enhance, although sometimes they can show very thin rim enhancement.

A

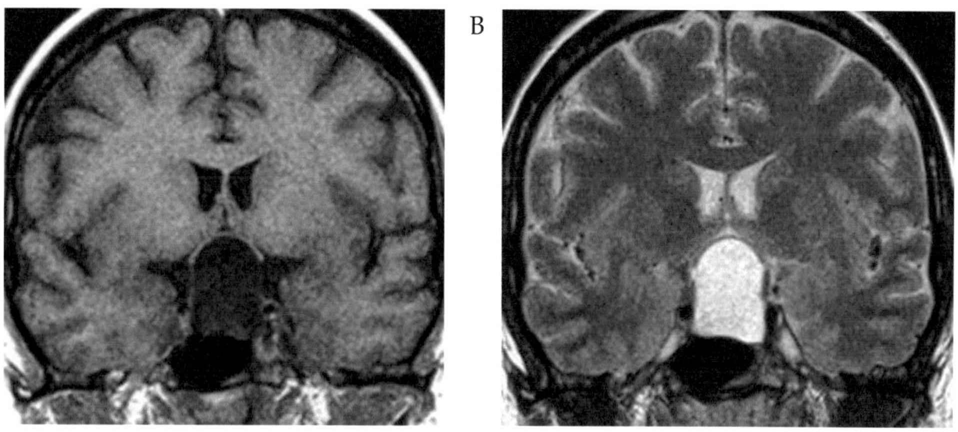


Fig. 16. MR imaging in coronal planes before contrast administration. A. T1-weighted image. B. T2-weighted image. Rathke's cleft cyst containing serous fluid - it is hypointense on T1 and hyperintense on T2-weighted image.

A

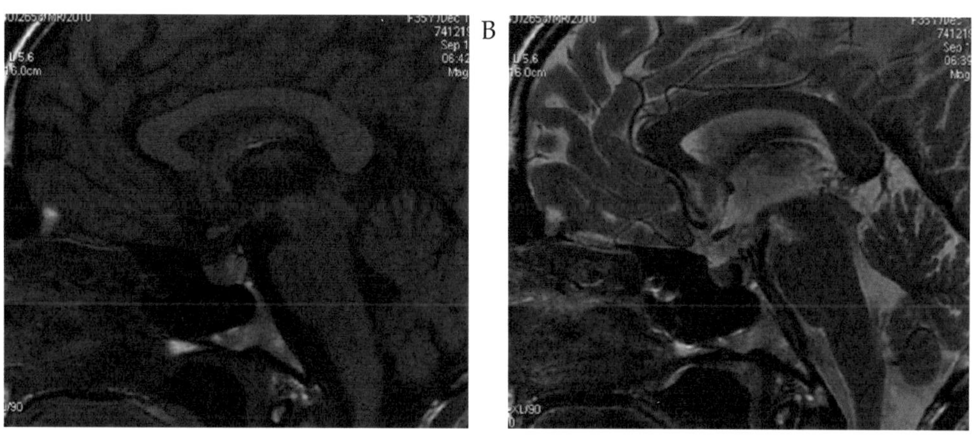


Fig. 17. MR imaging in sagittal planes before contrast administration. A. T1-weighted image. B. T2-weighted image. Rathke's cleft cyst containing mucoid fluid - it is hyperintense on T1 and hypointense on T2-weighted image.

Other cysts located in the sellar and parasellar region include: arachnoid, dermoid, epidermoid and colloid cysts (Bladowska et al., 2010c; Doerfler & Richter 2008).

### 4.3 Meningiomas

Meningiomas of the sellar region (cavernous sinus, planum sphenoidale, diaphragm sellae and clinoid process) account for about 11% of all sellar and parasellar tumors and for 20-30% of all intracranial meningiomas (Doerfler & Richter 2008). They are slow-growing, usually benign tumors.

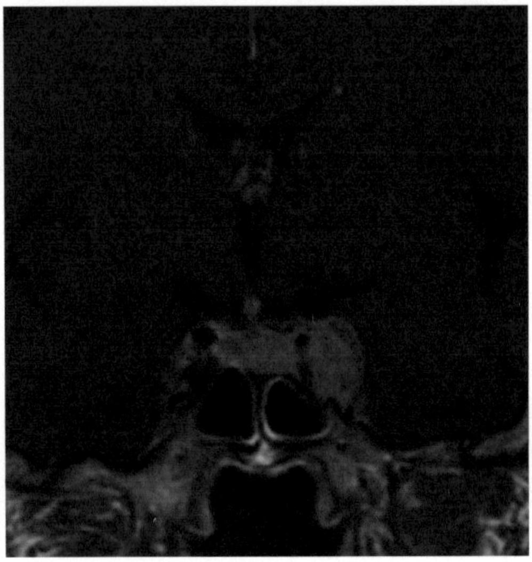

Fig. 18. T1-weighted coronal contrast-enhanced image. The meningioma of the left cavernous sinus is visible.

In MR imaging meningiomas are isointense compared to grey matter on T1-weighted images and isointense or slightly hyperintense on T2-weighted images. After contrast administration they reveal homogeneous enhancement (Fig.18). Often they present with characteristic so-called "dural tail sign", what can help in differential diagnosis, but it has to be stressed that the "dural tail sign" is a nonspecific feature and may also be visible in other intracranial tumors.

### 4.4 Other rare sellar and parasellar lesions

Rare primary neoplasm of the pituitary and sellar region include: melanoma, intrasellar meningioma, germinoma, choristoma, glioma and metastases (Elster 1993; Ruscalleda 2005). Inflammatory and infectious lesions of pituitary and sellar region include: abscess (Fig.19) (Bladowska et al., 2010d), sarcoidosis, cysticercosis, Langerhans cell histiocytosis, blastomycosis, Wegener granulomatosis, Tolosa-Hunt syndrome, lymphocytic adenohypophysitis, giant cell granuloma and tuberculosis (Elster 1993; Doerfler & Richter 2008).

A B

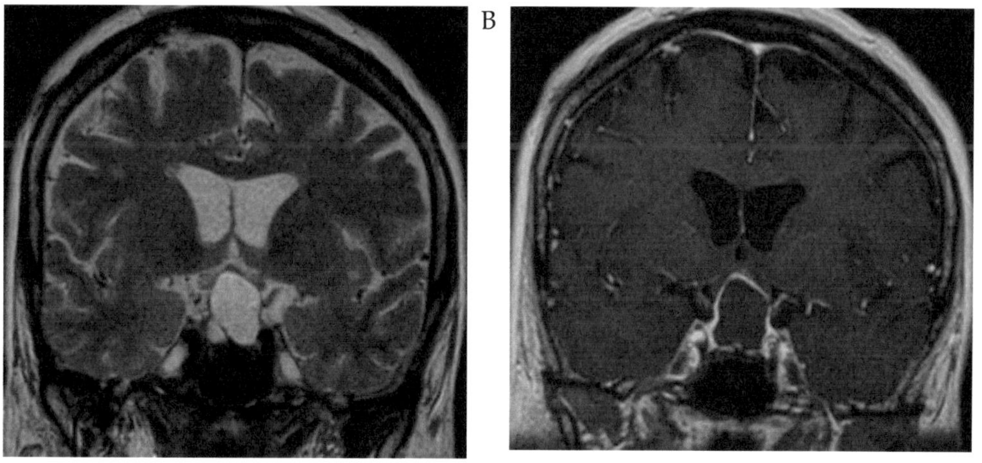

Fig. 19. MR imaging in coronal planes of the pituitary abscess. A. T2-weighted unenhanced image. B. T1-weighted contrast-enhanced image. There is characteristic strong rim enhancement visible.

## 5. Postoperative MR imaging of pituitary and sellar region – own experience

Post-surgical evaluation of the pituitary gland in MR is difficult because of a change in anatomical conditions. Interpretation of MR images taken after surgical therapy of pituitary tumors depends also on numerous other factors, including: size and expansion of a tumor before operation, type of surgical access, quality and volume of filling material and time of its resorption. Proper evaluation of post-surgical MR images is crucial for determination of completeness of the resection. Therefore neuro-radiologists face a responsible and difficult task of evaluation of structures present in the surgical area, and especially of differentiation of residual tumor from the implanted material and from post-surgical changes (fibrous and cicatrical), or even from a part of normal gland left at site (Bladowska et al., 2010a,b).

In general, the residual tumors could be differentiated from postoperative changes by means of location, characteristic signal intensity and enhancing pattern, which should be similar to those in the preoperative MR imaging of the tumor. The infundibulum tilt could be additional factor suggesting the presence of residual adenoma. The endocrine studies are very helpful in postoperative diagnosis of hormone-secreting residual pituitary adenomas and are regarded as a method of choice in postoperative management of these tumors. It is especially difficult to evaluate the effectiveness of the surgical treatment of the nonfunctioning pituitary tumors, these tumors require a postsurgical MR follow-up examinations.

The basic therapeutic method of pituitary tumors (apart from microprolactinoma) is surgery. Among several operation methods of the sellar region, the most frequently applied is the one with transnasal transsphenoidal approach. This method has widely forced out craniotomy and is now concerned the method of choice in the treatment of the majority of pituitary adenomas, both the hormonally active and inactive ones (Bladowska et al., 2010b).

A characteristic feature of transsphenoidal surgery is the necessity of applying different filling materials to obtain haemostasis, to fill the resection site within the sella, and to inhibit the outflow of the CSF (cerebrospinal fluid).

Filling materials are foreign or autogenic bodies that do not become vascularised. To sustain haemostasis, the following materials are used: oxidized cellulose (Oxycel or Surgicel), spongostan (Gelfoam), tissue glue (Tissucol or Beriplast), bone wax (to restrain bleeding from bone). Liquorrhoea requires a reconstructive operation of sella, with the use of autogenic fascia, lyophilisated dura mater or tissue glue. Next, the sella is sealed with a muscle or flakes of oxidized cellulose. To close the bottom of the sella, it is necessary to use a fragment of the collected cartilaginous septum from the nose, the vomer, or a silicon plate. To protect the postresection site and to reinforce the bottom of the sella, an autogenic fat graft is implanted in the sphenoid sinus. The graft is collected from the fatty tissue of the lateral part of the thigh or from the patient's abdomen (Bladowska et al., 2010b).

Application of the filling materials constitutes a considerable challenge in interpretation of the MR imaging results in patients who underwent surgery of the pituitary tumors. This can also lead to misdiagnosis. The knowledge of MR characteristics of the implanted materials is very important in postoperative diagnosis of pituitary tumors and may help to discriminate between tumorous and non-tumorous involvement of the sellar region (Bladowska et al., 2010b).

In the MRI examination, on T1-weighted images, Surgicel (Oxycel) is represented by a heterogeneous structure with a regular, oval shape, low signal intensity, surrounded by a hyperintense rim. Examinations performed in the first days after the procedure, frequently reveal the presence of small air bubbles closed in the strips of Surgicel, in the hypointense central part of the filling material (Bladowska et al., 2010b; Bonneville et al., 2003).

Spongostan (gelfoam) is represented in the MRI examination by an intrasellar mass of signal intensity similar to that of the grey matter. In rare cases, spongostan may produce a heterogeneous high signal caused most probably by the presence of methemoglobin (Bladowska et al., 2010b; Bonneville et al., 2003).

The similarity between signal intensity of the filling material, of the anterior pituitary lobe, and of a potential residual tumour often makes it difficult to interpret the image in an unequivocal way and to carry out a correct differential diagnosis. However, according to T. Kilic et al., spongostan and Surgicel (Oxycel) may be recognised only on an early performed MRI, i.e. within 24–48 hours after the procedure, because afterwards, the materials begin to undergo a progressive degeneration and their radiological identification becomes harder (Kilic et al., 2001). E. Steiner et al reported that these materials are normally recognisable on MRI for up to 3–6 months after the procedure (Steiner et al., 1992). Our studies showed that haemostatic materials may be identified only in the early postoperative period - in own material is was 1 month (Fig.20) (Bladowska et al., 2010b).

After contrast administration, the central part of the haemostatic material remained hypointense, with peripheral rim of enhancement. This peripheral enhancement is caused by granulation tissue forming around the implanted material. Filling materials undergo changes which surely inhibit their identification. It should be underscored that a hypointense mass with peripheral enhancement after contrast administration is not characteristic for the filling material only. It may also correspond to the presence of a fluid

A B

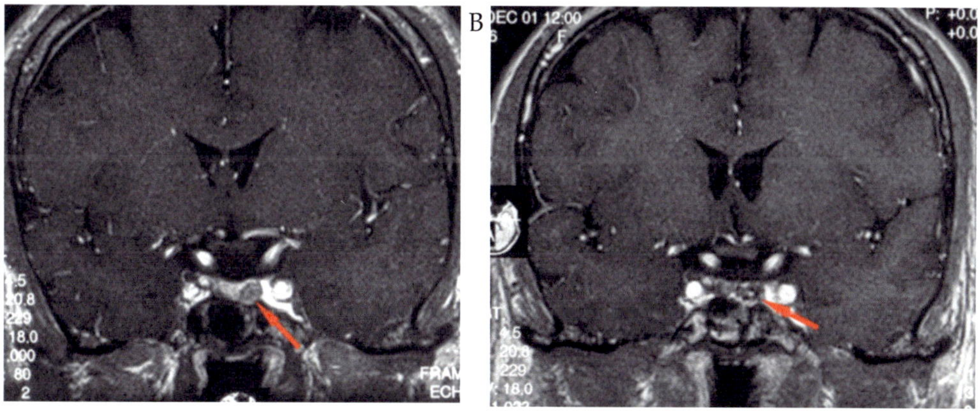

Fig. 20. T1-weighted contrast-enhanced coronal images. A. Before operation – on the left side of the pituitary the microadenoma is visible (arrow). B. Follow-up MRI performed 1 month after surgery – there is haemostatic material implanted into the operation site (arrow).

cistern, regions of necrosis within the tumor or cicatrical fibrous tissue with granulation around it (Bladowska et al., 2010b; Bonneville et al., 2003).

In our own material, as much as 85.61% of the patients had their first postoperative MRI examination performed after 3 months following the procedure, and only 14.39% of the studied individuals (20 patients) – during the first 3 months. There were no examinations carried out within 24–48 hours from the procedure. When we consider the date of MRI examinations and the fast degeneration of the filling material, it is then easy to explain the fact why the haemostatic material was identified in only two patients of the studied group.

The analysis of the conducted examinations revealed that the implanted autogenic fat and muscle with fascia, located in the lumen of the sphenoid sinus, can be observed on MRI for much longer (Bladowska et al., 2010b).

Fatty tissue is not too difficult to identify, as it provides a characteristic signal of high intensity on T1-weighted images (Fig.21). There were reported cases of residual fatty material present in the sphenoidal sinus examined at 1–2 years after the procedure or even 3–4 years afterwards. However, according to our assessments, the implanted fat may remain in place for much longer. The volume of the implanted fat influences the duration of its presence on MRI. Normally, the adipose tissue implanted in larger amounts (in case of macroadenoma resection) retains for much longer than the small amount of that material (implanted after microadenoma resection), absorbed within 9–12 months.

As compared to other filling materials, identification of the fatty tissue in the MRI examination is easy thanks to the characteristic high signal intensity produced by the material, its longer persistence, but also the absence of adjacent contrast-enhanced areas formed by the granulation tissue.

In the studied material, the implanted fatty tissue was identified in as many as 86 patients after pituitary tumour surgery. In the remaining 12 patients, who according to surgical reports were implanted fatty filling material, it was impossible to find that material on MRI. No fatty tissue found in these patients may result from a small amount of the implanted material, from its fast absorption, as well as from a longer postoperative time to MRI examination.

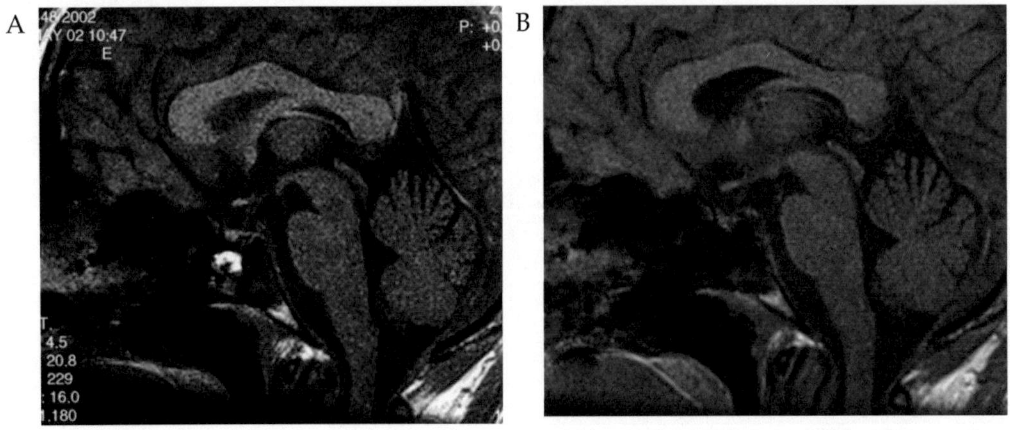


Fig. 21. T1-weighted unenhanced sagittal images. A. MRI performed 10 months after transsphenoidal operation reveals the implanted fatty material inside the sphenoid sinus – it presents with high signal intensity. B. Follow-up MRI performed 23 months after surgery – there is no implanted material visible.

The earliest total absorption of the fatty material was observed 11 months after the procedure. In most of the cases, residues of the adipose tissue were present for a long time, for even up to 112 months (nearly 10 years) after the procedure, while in one patient, there was a large amount of the fatty material still present in the lumen of the sphenoidal sinus after 348 months (29 years) (Bladowska et al., 2010b).

In 2 patients, it was possible to visualise the implanted titanium mesh (Fig.22). On MRI, the titanium mesh was represented by a linear area producing no signal and located in the bottom of the sella (Bladowska et al., 2010b).

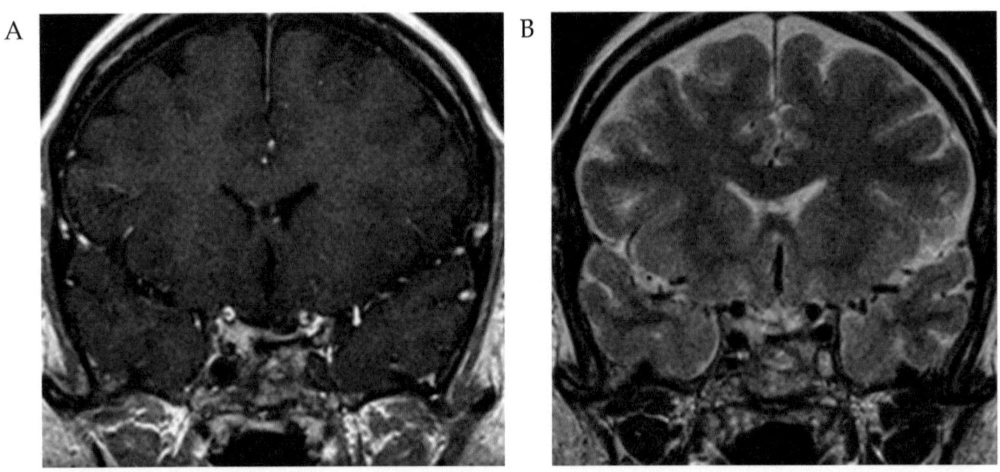


Fig. 22. MR imaging of implanted titanium mesh. A. T1-weighted coronal image. B. T2-weighted coronal image. A linear area producing no signal and located in the bottom of the sella is visible.

In 3 individuals, an implanted muscle with fascia was identified. It was represented by a round, isointense structure, filling nearly the whole sphenoidal sinus on T1-weighted MRI images. After intravenous contrast administration, the structure was becoming slightly enhanced in its peripheral part, with a central round area of lower signal intensity (Fig.23a). Such an image of the implanted muscle was found in 2 patients after 4 months following the procedure, and in 1 patient after 5 months from surgery. The follow-up MRIs (beginning approx. from the 12$^{th}$ postoperative month) were revealing a gradual change in the image of that material. After contrast administration, the previously distinct border between the enhanced peripheral part and the central hypointense part of the implanted muscle became indistinct. In further MRI examinations, performed approx. 25 months after surgery or later, the structure present in the lumen of the sphenoidal sinus remained hypointense after contrast administration. Without the analysis of previous images and the knowledge of patient's history, the correct diagnosis of that mass on T1-weighted images was impossible (especially its differentiation from e.g. fluid cistern). The implanted muscle with fascia produced a very characteristic and almost stable image in T2-weighted sequence (Fig.23b), for at least 31 months following the procedure. In the T2-weighted sequence, the material is represented by a hyperintense mass with a linear structure, of a very low signal intensity, corresponding to fascia (Fig.23b). It should also be pointed out that fascia was not identified on T1-weighted images (Fig.23a) (Bladowska et al., 2010b, 2011).

A B

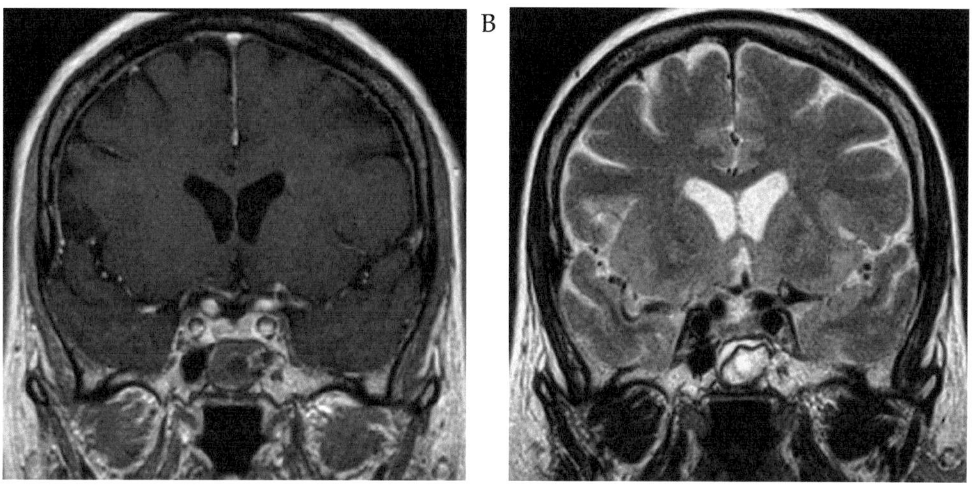

Fig. 23. MR imaging of muscle with fascia implanted into the sphenoid sinus. A. T1-weighted enhanced coronal image. B. T2- weighted unenhanced coronal image - the linear structure, of a very low signal intensity, corresponding to fascia is very well visible.

The final diagnosis and evaluation of the surgical completeness on the basis of the performed MRI is often equivocal, in spite of the presence of the above mentioned criteria.

It is especially hard to evaluate the effectiveness of the surgical treatment of the hormonally inactive tumors on the basis of the MRI examination results and their interpretation only. These tumors require a postsurgical endocrinological and MRI follow-up.

Follow-up of abnormal structures present in the postsurgical area may allow for their verification. If in the following examinations there is a complete absorption of the focal lesion, this excludes the presence of a residual tumor and indicates to the filling material or postoperative changes.

If the size and volume of the pathological structure increases, this points to the presence of a residual tumor. On the other hand, it should be remembered that pituitary tumors grow slowly, so in a long-term follow-up, the tumor may seem stable, which does not facilitate the final diagnosis in unclear cases of hormonally inactive tumors.

As mentioned above, the transsphenoidal approach is currently the method of choice in treatment of most of pituitary tumors. There are characteristic changes inside the sphenoid sinus after the surgery (Connor & Deasy, 2002). MRI findings of sphenoid sinus filling (opacification) are present in approximately 37% of examinations performed more than 12 months after transsphenoidal surgery. The contrast enhancement at the margins of the sphenoid sinus, called as Rodriguez's changes (Fig.24), is always apparent in cases of hypervascularized and swollen mucosa (Rodriguez et al., 1996) and could persist even 10 years after surgery.

A B

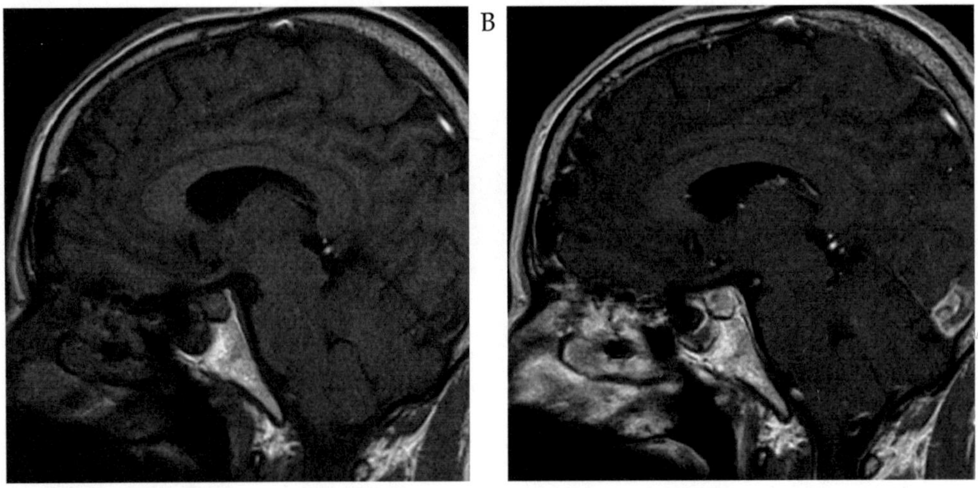

Fig. 24. MR imaging of Rodriguez's changes, T1-weighted sagittal images: unenhanced (A), contrast-enhanced (B). There are hypointense masses inside the sphenoid sinus, which show the characteristic rim contrast enhancement.

The special attention should be also paid to usefulness of T2-weighted images in assessment of postoperative sella and sellar region. T2-weighted images may help to discriminate between tumorous and non-tumorous involvement of the postoperative sella and the sphenoid sinus especially in cases, in which the signal intensity and enhancement pattern of pituitary gland and tumor are the same on T1-weighted images. T2-weighted images are also very useful in the postoperative evaluation of the implanted muscle with fascia, especially during long term follow-up. The best protocol for the postoperative imaging after pituitary tumor resections should include both T1- and T2-weighted imaging, because T1- and T2-weighted images supplement each other in the postoperative examination of the sella and sellar region. However, in some cases T2 could replace post-contrast T1, especially in patients with high risk of Nephrogenic Systemic Fibrosis (NSF) (Bladowska et al., 2011).

## 6. Conclusion

Pituitary adenomas are common neoplasm, they account for 10-15% of all diagnosed intracranial tumors. The proper diagnosis and management of patients with pituitary lesions are of high importance in the clinical practice. Currently, MR is the method of choice for imaging of the pituitary gland and the parasellar area. MR imaging protocol of pituitary and sellar region including postoperative studies should consist of unenhanced T1- and T2-weighted images in coronal and sagittal planes, followed by T1-weighted images after contrast administration. Because of so many pathological changes with different clinical and radiological appearances of the lesions located in sellar and parasellar region, the precise knowledge of pituitary lesions is mandatory for the correct diagnosis and management of patients with pituitary diseases.

## 7. Acknowledgment

I would like to thank my dear husband Maciej, my lovely daughters Justynka and Hania, and my all family for the patience, they have given me during the time I was writing this chapter. I will use the words of Robert C. Martin:

"There is no greater treasure, nor any wealthier trove, than the company of my family, and the comfort of their love".

Joanna Bladowska

## 8. References

Arslan A., Karaarslan E., Dincer A. (1999) High intensity signal of the posterior pituitary. A study with horizontal direction of frequency-encoding and fat suppression MR techniques. *Acta Radiologica*, Vol. 40, (1999) pp. 142-145.

Bladowska J., Sokolska V., Czapiga E., Badowski R., Koźmińska U., Moroń K. (2004) Advances in diagnostics imaging of the pituitary and the parasellar region. *Advances in Clinical and Experimental Medicine*, Vol. 13, (2004) pp. 709-717.

Bladowska J, Sokolska V, Sozański T et al. (2010) Comparison of post-surgical MRI presentation of the pituitary gland and its hormonal function. *Polish Journal of Radiology*, Vol. 75, (2010) pp. 29-36.

Bladowska J, Bednarek-Tupikowska G, Sokolska V et al. (2010) MRI image characteristics of materials implanted at sellar region after transsphenoidal resection of pituitary tumours. *Polish Journal of Radiology*, Vol.75, (2010), pp. 46-54.

Bladowska J, Bednarek-Tupikowska G, Biel A, Sąsiadek M. (2010) Colloid cyst of the pituitary gland: Case report and literature review. *Polish Journal of Radiology*, Vol.75, (2010), pp. 92-97.

Bladowska J, Bednarek-Tupikowska G, Sokolska V, Czapiga E, Czapiga B, Sąsiadek M. (2010) Unusual presentation of recurrent pituitary abscess - a case report and literature review. *Neuroradiology Journal*, Vol.23, (2010), pp. 547-553.

Bladowska J, Biel A, Zimny A et al. (2011) Are the T2-weighted images more useful than T1-weighted contrast-enhanced images in assessment of postoperative sella and parasellar region? *Medical Science Monitor*, Vol. 17, no 10 (October 2011), pp. MT83-MT90.

Bonneville JF. (2000) Pituitary adenomas: value of MR imaging. *Journal of Radiology,* Vol.81, (2000), pp. 939-942.

Bonneville JF, Bonneville F, Schillo F, Cattin F, Jacquet G. (2003) Follow-up MRI after trans-sphenoidal surgery. *Journal of Neuroradiology,* Vol.30, (2003), pp. 268-279.

Bonneville JF, Bonneville F, Cattin F. (2005) Magnetic resonance imaging of pituitary adenomas. *European Radiology,* Vol. 15, (2005) pp. 543-548.

Boxerman JL, Rogg JM, Donahue JE et al. (2010) Preoperative MRI evaluation of pituitary macroadenoma: imaging features predictive of successful transsphenoidal surgery. *American Journal of Radiology AJR,* Vol.195, (2010), pp. 720-728.

Chernov MF., Kawamata T., Amano K. et al. (2009) Possible role of single-voxel $^{1}$H-MRS in differential diagnosis of suprasellar tumors. *Journal of Neurooncology,* Vol.91, (2009), pp. 191-198.

Connor SEJ. & Deasy NP. (2002) MRI appearances of the sphenoid sinus at the late follow-up of trans-sphenoidal surgery for pituitary macroadenoma. *Australasian Radiology,* Vol.46, (2002), pp. 33-40.

Daly AF, Tichomirowa MA, Beckers A. (2009) The epidemiology and genetics of pituitary adenomas. *Best Practice & Research Clinical Endocrinology & Metabolism;* Vol.23, (2009), pp. 543–554.

Doerfler A. & Richter G. (2008) Lesions within and around the pituitary. *Clinical Neuroradiology;* Vol.18, (2008), pp. 5-18.

Elster A.D. (1993) Modern imaging of the pituitary. *Radiology,* Vol.187, (1993), pp. 1-14.

Elster A.D., Chen M.Y.M., Williams D.W., Key L.L. (1990) Pituitary gland: MR imaging of physiologic hypertrophy in adolescence. *Radiology,* Vol.174, (1990), pp. 681-685.

Elster A.D., Sanders T.G., Vines F.S., Chen M.Y.M. (1991) Size and shape of the pituitary gland during pregnancy and post partum: measurement with MR imaging. *Radiology,* Vol.181, (1991), pp. 531-535.

Evanson J. (2002) Imaging the pituitary gland. *Imaging,* Vol.14, (2002), pp. 93-102.

Kilic T, Ekinci G, Seker A et al. (2001). Determining optimal MRI follow-up after transsphenoidal surgery for pituitary adenomas: scan at 24 hours postsurgery provides reliable information. *Acta Neurochirurgica* (Wien), Vol.143, (2001), pp. 1103–26.

Rodriguez O, Mateos B, de la Pedraja R et al. (1996) Postoperative follow-up of pituitary adenomas after transsphenoidal resection: MRI and clinical correlation. *Neuroradiology,* Vol.38, (1996), pp. 747–54.

Ruscalleda J. (2005) Imaging of parasellar lesions. *European Radiology,* Vol.15, (2005), pp. 549-559.

Steiner E, Knosp E, Herold ChJ et al (1992): Pituitary adenomas: Findings of postoperative MR imaging. *Radiology,* Vol.185, (1992), pp. 521–27.

# 3

# Functioning Pituitary Adenoma

Mahdi Sharif-Alhoseini[1], Edward R. Laws[2] and Vafa Rahimi-Movaghar[3,4]
[1]*Sina Trauma and Surgery Research Center, Tehran University of Medical Sciences, Tehran,*
[2]*Department of Neurosurgery, Brigham & Women's Hospital, Harvard Medical School, Boston, Massachusetts,*
[3]*Sina Trauma and Surgery Research Center, Department of Neurosurgery, Tehran University of Medical Sciences, Tehran,*
[4]*Research Centre for Neural Repair, University of Tehran, Tehran,*
[1,3,4]*Iran*
[2]*USA*

## 1. Introduction

Pituitary adenomas are typically benign, slow-growing tumors that arise from cells in the pituitary gland. Those are classified based on secretory products (1). The functioning (endocrine-active) tumors include almost 70% of pituitary tumors which produce 1 or 2 hormones that are measurable in the serum and cause definite clinical syndromes that are classified based on their secretory product(s). Non-functioning adenomas are endocrine-inactive tumors (2). Because of the physiologic effects of excess hormones, functioning tumors usually present earlier than non-functioning adenomas (3). On the other hand, mass effect from large pituitary adenomas (often due to endocrine-inactive tumors) may lead to pressure symptoms such as headaches, visual field defects (typically loss of peripheral vision), cranial nerve deficits, hypopituitarism (compression of normal pituitary gland), pituitary apoplexy (sudden bleeding or infarction from outgrowing tumor blood supply), or stalk dysfunction (4). Compression of pituitary stalk is termed "stalk effect" which can cause a mild elevation in prolactin, and must be differentiated from a prolactinoma (5).

The purpose of this chapter is to review all types of functioning pituitary adenoma (prolactin, ACTH, GH, TSH, LH and FSH secreting) from studies indexed in PubMed. We describe the symptoms, epidemiology, diagnosis, management, outcome and complications of each.

## 2. Prolactinoma

This type of pituitary adenoma arises from neoplastic transformation of anterior pituitary lactotrophs and produces an excessive amount of hormone prolactin. A prolactinoma is the most common cause of chronic hyperprolactinemia once pregnancy, primary hypothyroidism, and drugs that elevate serum prolactin levels have been excluded (6).

### 2.1 Symptoms

In female patients, even small prolactinomas can cause irregular menstrual periods or complete loss of menses. Higher prolactin levels lead to galactorrhea in women, whereas men may experience gynecomastia. In male patients, altered spermatogenesis with oligospermia and infertility may be found; galactorrhea and gynaecomastia are much less frequent. Hypogonadism, reduced libido and infertility are the most frequent symptoms in both genders. Patients can also present with osteopenia and osteoporosis (due to estrogen and testosterone deficiency, not due to the elevated prolactin itself). Large prolactinomas, more commonly found in men, may cause mass effect from the tumor (5-9).

### 2.2 Epidemiology

The estimated prevalence of prolactinoma is 100 per million adults (10). Prolactinomas are the most common hormone-secreting pituitary tumors, representing approximately 40% of all pituitary tumors (8, 11, 12). Recent data show a high prevalence of prolactinoma in the general population, 3-5 times more than the previously reported ones (13). The incidence of prolactinomas varies with age and sex; these tumors occur with the highest frequency in women aged 20–50 years, at which point the ratio between the sexes is estimated to be 10:1. In adults aged >60 years, prolactinomas occur with a similar frequency in both sexes (12). Men generally have macroadenomas (≥10mm diameter) whereas women generally have microadenomas (<10mm) (6, 13, 14). The mean age at diagnosis is 10 years greater in men. This delay possibly accounts for their greater incidence of macroprolactinomas with visual field defects and hypopituitarism at first presentation (15).

### 2.3 Diagnosis

A serum prolactin level is acquired in response to a specific presentation, including symptoms of hyperprolactinemia (such as amenorrhea and galactorrhea) it may also be an integral part of an infertility assessment. An initial level above the normal range should be followed by a repeat level from a blood sample drawn in the morning with the patient in a fasting state. When hyperprolactinemia is confirmed, a cause for the disorder needs to be sought. This involves a careful history and examination, followed by laboratory tests and diagnostic imaging of the sella turcica. If serum prolactin levels are above 200 μg/L, a prolactinoma is almost certainly the underlying cause, but if levels are lower, the differential diagnoses include pregnancy, treatment with drugs (such as neuroleptics) that reduce dopaminergic effects on the pituitary, compression of the pituitary stalk by other pathology, primary hypothyroidism, renal failure, cirrhosis, chest wall lesions, or idiopathic hyperprolactinemia. In the absence of such causes, radiologic imaging of the sella turcica is necessary to establish whether a prolactinoma or other lesions are present (4, 6, 16).

### 2.4 Management

The main purpose of treating prolactinomas, both micro- and macroprolactinomas, are to suppress excess hormone secretion and its clinical effects, to remove the tumor mass, and to prevent disease return or progression (16, 17). If there is no indication for therapy (such as amenorrhea, infertility or bothersome galactorrhea), microadenomas may be followed conservatively, and regular follow-up with serial prolactin measurements and pituitary imaging should be organized (6, 16). Most prolactinomas can be effectively treated with dopaminergic drugs as primary management. For most patients, medical therapy produces normalization of prolactin secretion, gonadal function, and considerable tumor shrinkage in the majority (16). The most commonly used dopamine agonists are bromocriptine, cabergoline (ergot derivatives) as well as quinagolide (a non-ergot derivative) (4, 18). Bromocriptine ($D_2$ receptor agonist and $D_1$ receptor antagonist) is the oldest drug for medical treatment of prolactinomas, and normalizes prolactin levels in 80-90% of microprolactinomas and 70% of macroprolactinomas. Tumor-mass shrinkage and improvement of visual-field deficits are commonly achieved in macroprolactinomas. Bromocriptine frequently can cause several side effects such as nausea, vomiting, postural hypotension, headache and dizziness (12). Cabergoline (a selective $D_2$ receptor agonist) is very effective and well tolerated in more than 90% of the patients with either microprolactinomas or macroprolactinomas. Cabergoline treatment also induces tumor shrinkage in most macroprolactinomas. If patients have not previously been treated with other dopamine agonists, tumor shrinkage is more evident (17). When comparing the plasma half-life, efficacy and tolerability of these drugs, cabergoline seems to have the most favorable profile, followed by quinagolide (16). As a well tolerated and effective therapy and a simple dosing regimen, quinagolide (selective D2 receptor agonist) can also be considered a first-line therapy in the treatment of hyperprolactinaemia (19). Pergolide (a D1 and D2 agonist) normalizes prolactin excess and reduces tumor size in recently diagnosed patients with macroprolactinomas with a potency of about 100-fold that of bromocriptine (20). However pergolide as approved treatment for prolactinomas was withdrawn in 2007 because of adverse effects on cardiac valves (12).

If prolactin levels are well controlled with dopamine agonist therapy, gradual tapering of the dose to the lowest effective amount is recommended, and in some cases medication can be stopped after several years. Evidence to date suggests that cabergoline and quinagolide appear to have a good safety profile for women who wish to conceive, but hard evidence proving that dopamine agonists do not provoke congenital malformations when taken during early pregnancy is currently only available for bromocriptine. Once pregnant, dopamine agonist therapy should be immediately stopped, unless the growth of a macroprolactinoma or pressure symptoms is likely to occur (4, 16). Hyperprolactinemia may recur after dopamine agonist withdrawal in a considerable proportion of patients. The probability of successful treatment was highest when cabergoline was used for at least two years (21).

Surgery is generally used as second-line treatment in prolactinomas (22). Transsphenoidal surgery is an alternative for patients who are intolerant of or resistant to dopamine agonists or when hyperprolactinemia is caused by non-prolactin-secreting tumors compressing the pituitary stalk (4).

Because pituitary adenomas respond well to radiation, radiotherapy has been a part of their management for the past three decades (23). Radiotherapy is given if both pharmacologic therapy and surgery fail (4, 16). However, Sasaki et al. reported that the local control rate for secreting adenomas by radiotherapy is unsatisfactory (23).

Gamma knife radiosurgery can be offered as a safe and effective treatment option especially for those patients with recurrent or residual pituitary adenoma after surgical removal. The tumor control rate after gamma knife radiosurgery for pituitary adenomas is equivalent to fractionated radiation therapy (24).

Some experimental treatments have been attempted, such as somatostatin analogues, hybrid molecules (both somatostatin and a dopamine agonist in a single molecule), selective estrogen receptor modulators, prolactin-receptor antagonists, and temozolomide are utilized in selected case reports or in trial settings. These have not yet been included in standard medical practice (12).

### 2.5 Outcome

The ultimate goal of therapy for prolactinomas is restoration or achievement of eugonadism through the normalization of hyperprolactinemia and control of tumor mass (11). Medical and surgical therapies generally have excellent results, and most prolactinomas are well controlled or even cured in some cases (19). Dopamine agonists are the preferred therapy for prolactinomas because of the risk of recurrent hyperprolactinemia that accompanies transsphenoidal surgery (25, 26). Dopamine agonists are the first line of therapy for macroprolactinomas, resulting in normalizing prolactin levels in 85%, inducing tumor shrinkage in 57%, and long-term remission rates in 22% of the patients (11, 27).

Surgery should be reserved for patients with dopamine agonist resistance or intolerance. Success rates after surgical treatment of microadenomas range from 73–90% and 30–50% for macroadenomas, with little morbidity and near zero mortality (28). However, subsequent relapse is possible in up to 20% of the cases (22). Surgical outcomes are highly dependent upon the expertise and experience of the neurosurgeon (11, 22).

Following radiotherapy the prevalence of subsequent hypopituitarism is high; therefore, this therapy should be carefully considered, and rather be indicated for mass control than for hyperprolactinemia (27).

Overall, patients with pituitary adenoma treated with surgery and radiotherapy have an increased risk of cerebrovascular motrtality compared to the general population, which mirrors the increased incidence of stroke (29).

### 2.6 Complications

As mentioned in the symptoms section, prolactinomas left untreated may lead to various complications. In both women and men, prolactinoma can cause reduced libido, infertility and osteoporosis. Women with prolactinoma may experience complications during pregnancy. A woman who has a large prolactinoma and becomes pregnant may experience additional pituitary growth and associated mass effect. Prolactinoma may also lead to impaired glucose tolerance and diabetes. If tumor grows large enough, prolactinoma may cause visual loss, headache and hypopituitarism. Disturbances of the haemostatic system and dyslipidemia may lead to excess mortality in patients with prolactinoma (5-9, 30, 31).

## 3. ACTH secreting PA

Approximately 80% of the cases of Cushing's syndrome are due to the excessive secretion of adrenocorticotropic hormone (ACTH). This is usually (60-80%) due to a pituitary corticotroph adenoma and is defined as Cushing's disease (2, 32).

### 3.1 Symptoms

Cushing's syndrome refers to clinical manifestations induced by chronic exposure to excess glucocorticoids. The most common symptom of glucocorticoid excess is centripetal fat deposition which is frequently the initial symptom of the patient.

Fat accumulates in the face as well as supraclavicular and dorsocervical fat pads, resulting in a typical moon face and buffalo hump, which is most often accompanied by facial plethora. Fat also accumulates over the thorax and the abdomen, which becomes protuberant (33).

Other symptoms and signs include obesity; protein-wasting features such as skin thinning, large and purple abdominal striae, multiple ecchymotic lesions or purpura generated by minimal trauma, lower limb edema, spontaneous ruptures of tendons, slow healing of minor wounds, muscle atrophy, particularly in the lower limbs; bone wasting such as osteoporosis, pathological fractures, kyphosis and loss of height (34, 35); impaired protection mechanism against infections (36); high blood pressure and cardiovascular complications (37, 38); hirsutism; gonadal dysfunction (39); psychic disturbances such as anxiety, irritability, sleep disorders, depression, maniac disorders, delusions and/or hallucinations (40); and decreased short-term memory and cognition (41).

### 3.2 Epidemiology

The prevalence of Cushing's disease is approximately 40 per million. ACTH-producing adenomas comprise 10-20% of pituitary adenomas (42). Cushing's disease is nine times more common in women than men(2).

### 3.3 Diagnosis

The clinical history is important to assess the general impact of hypercortisolism on organs and systems as well as to guide suspicion toward more aggressive entities such as the ectopic ACTH syndrome or to detect an iatrogenic etiology of Cushing's syndrome (43). Initial diagnosis is performed using tests such as urinary free cortisol, nocturnal salivary cortisol and 1 mg dexamethasone suppression that are sensitive but not specific, and still require established assessment criteria(44). A dexamethasone- corticotrophin releasing hormone (CRH) test can discriminate between Cushing's syndrome and pseudo-Cushing's syndrome. If ACTH is elevated, combinations of high-dose dexamethasone tests, CRH/desmopressin tests, and pituitary magnetic resonance imaging can indicate a pituitary source. Discrimination from an ectopic ACTH tumor often requires inferior petrosal sinus sampling to confirm the source of ACTH. If ACTH is low, adrenal computed tomography will identify the adrenal lesion(s) implicated. Some cortisol-producing adrenal tumors or, more frequently, bilateral macronodular hyperplasia, are under the control of aberrant membrane hormone receptors, or the altered activity of ectopic receptors (43-46). Sophisticated imaging and isotopic techniques play a significant role in locating the source of ACTH in ectopic syndromes but are not always effective. In general, biochemical and imaging tests should be combined in order to assess different mechanisms and perspectives of the syndrome. Rigorous methodology is essential to obtain accurate results, allowing a correct diagnosis and in improving therapeutic performance in this devastating disease (43).

### 3.4 Management

The best treatment option for Cushing's disease is when the responsible corticotroph adenoma can be entirely removed surgically by the trans-sphenoidal approach, with sufficient skill to preserve normal anterior pituitary function (32, 46). This induces remission in approximately 80% of the patients, but long-term relapse occurs in up to 30% of these cases (45). The choice of second-line therapy remains controversial (46). Repeat surgery can be successful when residual tumor is detectable on magnetic resonance imaging; however, it carries a high risk of hypopituitarism. The histological pseudocapsule of a pituitary adenoma is a layer of compressed normal anterior lobe that surrounds the adenoma and can be used during surgery to identify and guide the removal of the tumor. With this approach, the overall remission rate is high and the rate of complications is low (47). Radiotherapy combined with ketoconazole or radiosurgery was recently found effective, but a longer-term evaluation of hypopituitarism and brain function is required. As soon as residual tumor progresses, surgery and radiotherapy should be initiated. Various drugs which inhibit steroid synthesis (ketoconazole, metyrapone, aminoglutethimide, mitotane) are sometimes temporarily effective for rapidly controlling hypercortisolism either in preparation for surgery, after the unsuccessful removal of the etiologic tumor, or while awaiting the full effect of radiotherapy or more definitive therapy (45). Other modes of radiotherapy (heavy particles, stereotactic radiosurgery with gamma knife) are limited to specialized centers. Despite initial enthusiasm for gamma knife (48), a relapse rate of up to 20% has been reported following treatment. It may, however, be more rapid than conventional radiotherapy in onset of lowering cortisol levels (49).

### 3.5 Outcome

The long-term follow-up of patients treated for Cushing's disease should include the adequate replacement of glucocorticoids and other hormones, treatment of osteoporosis, and detection of long-term relapse of Cushing's disease (45). Following pituitary surgery, careful ongoing expert endocrine assessment is mandatory, as the incidence of relapse increases with time and also with the increasing rigor of the endocrine evaluation. (50).

### 3.6 Complications

Today, cardiovascular and psychiatric co-morbidities still remain the major life-threatening complication. The final prognostic criterion for Cushing's syndrome lies in the severity of the hypercortisolism and the aggressiveness of the responsible tumor (37, 46). Bone wasting results in generalized osteoporosis. The prevalence of bone demineralisation assessed by bone mineral density using dual energy X-ray absorptiometry is about 40% (51). Compression fractures of the spine are evident on plain radiographs in about 20% - 80% of the patients, depending on the studies, and almost half the patients complain about backache. Kyphosis and loss of height, sometimes dramatic, are frequent. Pathological fractures can occur elsewhere, particularly in the ribs, feet and pelvis (36). Transient features of brain atrophy can disappear after cure (52). Impaired quality of life may persist years after controlling hypercortisolism (53).

## 4. GH secreting PA

Excessive secretion of growth hormone (GH) is responsible for acromegaly (54). This disease is almost always due to a GH-secreting pituitary adenoma. It is distinguished by a gradual progressively acquired somatic disfigurement (primarily involving the face and extremities) and leads to acromegaly: a disorder of disproportionate tissue, skeletal, and organ growth (55, 56).

### 4.1 Symptoms

Because of the insidious onset and slow progression, acromegaly is frequently diagnosed from four to more than ten years after its onset (57). Patients usually display coarsened facial appearance, acral enlargement, increased skin thickness and soft tissue hyperplasia. Other manifestations include increased sweating, goiter, joint involvement, carpal tunnel syndrome, visual abnormalities, headache, colon polyps, sleep apnea, reproductive disorders, metabolic disturbances (hypertriglyceridemia, reduced insulin sensitivity), and cardiovascular disease (cardiac hypertrophy, hypertension, arrhythmias, and cardiomyopathy) (57-59).

### 4.2 Epidemiology

The prevalence is estimated to be 40-130 per million inhabitants, with 3-4 new cases per million populations per year (55, 58). It is most often diagnosed in middle-aged adults (average age 40 years). Men and women are equally affected (57).

### 4.3 Diagnosis

The measurement of fasting or random GH and of Insulin-like Growth Factor 1 (IGF-1) are baseline biochemical criteria for the diagnosis of acromegaly. A random GH level lower than 0.4 µg/l and an IGF-1 value in the age- and sex-matched normal range exclude the diagnosis of acromegaly. When these two parameters are dissonant, a 75 gram oral glucose tolerance test (OGTT) should be performed: a fall of serum GH to 1 µg/l or less within two hours will exclude acromegaly (60, 61).

Measurement of circulating GH-releasing hormone (GHRH) is the preferred test for the differential diagnosis between GH-secreting pituitary adenoma and ectopic GHRH secretion. Stimulatory tests (thyroid releasing hormone (TRH) stimulation test or gonadotropin releasing hormone (GnRH) stimulation test) provide no advantage over OGTT, and their use is not recommended for diagnosis (58).

Acromegaly is caused by an adenoma of the pituitary gland in more than 98% of all patients. The size of the tumor and its expansion should be documented by MRI. If the tumor expands into the suprasellar space and/or laterally beyond the cavernous sinus, an ophthalmological assessment is suggested to determine the possible impairment of the visual field and function of oculomotor nerves (58).

### 4.4 Management

The goal of treatment is to relieve symptoms, to obtain control of local tumor mass, and to reduce morbidity and mortality. Treatment options include surgery, medical therapy and radiotherapy. Transsphenoidal surgery is the first choice of treatment when a definitive cure can be achieved, mainly in the cases of microadenomas and when decompression of surrounding structures (optic chiasm, ophthalmic motor nerves) is indicated. This treatment is the first-line therapy except when the macroadenoma is giant or if surgery is contra-indicated. Primary medical therapy should be conducted in patients bearing macroadenomas with significant lateral extension. In addition, preoperative primary medical therapy may result in tumor shrinkage, facilitating tumor resection, and may reduce preoperative complications due to GH excess. Within the spectrum of medical therapy, long-acting somatostatin analogues (somatostatins) are considered as primary therapy. Treatment with somatostatins results in GH control in about 60% of the cases. Somatostatins also induce tumor contraction in 30-50% of the patients, most effectively when applied as first-line treatment. Prolonged treatment with somatostatins is safe and well tolerated. Octreotide and lanreotide (two currently available somatostatins) appear to have equal effectiveness. In patients with suboptimal clinical and biochemical response to somatostatins, combination therapy with dopamine receptor agonists or pegvisomant (a new GH-receptor antagonist) typically leads to effective disease control. New developments in the medical therapy of acromegaly include the universal somatostatin receptor agonist pasireotide, and chimerical compounds that interact with both somatostatin and dopamine receptors with synergizing effects on GH secretion (54, 58, 62, 63).

If surgery fails, medical therapy should be started or reinstated. Dopaminergic drugs might be considered for a small group of patients with mildly elevated GH/IGF-1 levels or harboring GH-prolactin co-secreting adenomas (64, 65). The use of radiotherapy (fractionated, or by gamma-knife) appears to be justified as a treatment of last resort in patients with tumors progressively growing and unresponsive to somatostatins, and in a small group of patients who bear aggressive pituitary adenomas invasive of local structures including the cavernous sinus and even the temporal lobes. These tumors occur more frequently in younger patients, for whom the concerns about radiation-dependent hypopituitarism and second tumor formation are higher. Therefore several considerations must be taken into account when choosing an individualized treatment program for each patient (63, 66).

### 4.5 Outcome

Rheumatologic, cardiovascular, respiratory and metabolic consequences are major factors that determine the prognosis (55). The control of GH and IGF-1 secretion is the main goal of treatment, since normalization of these two parameters is the most significant determinant of reversing the increased mortality rate of the patients. The outcome of transsphenoidal surgery is far better for microadenomas (80-90%) than for macroadenomas (less than 50%), which unfortunately represent more than 70% of all GH-secreting pituitary tumors. Therefore, pituitary surgery is the first line treatment for microadenomas (58). Indeed, survival in acromegaly is restored to that observed in the general population after correction of GH/IGF-1 hypersecretion, while morbidity (obstructive sleep apnea, carpal tunnel syndrome, cardiac dysfunction, and diabetes mellitus) is markedly improved by lowering IGF-1 levels(67).

### 4.6 Complications

Acromegaly is a slowly progressive disease characterized by a 30% increase of mortality rate for cardiovascular disease (atherosclerosis, cardiomyopathy), respiratory complications, arthrosis and malignancies. Patients with acromegaly display an enhanced mortality rate, cardiovascular disease represents the cause of death in 60%, respiratory disease in 25% and malignancies in 15% of the cases. High GH levels, high blood pressure and heart disease represent the major negative survival determinants in acromegaly, whereas symptom duration, diabetes mellitus and cancer play a minor role in determining mortality (54, 58). If the condition is untreated, enhanced mortality due to cardiovascular, cerebrovascular, and pulmonary dysfunction is associated with a 30% decrease in life span (56).

## 5. TSH secreting PA

Thyroid stimulating hormone (TSH) secreting pituitary adenomas are a rare cause of secondary or central hyperthyroidism (68, 69). The pathogenesis of TSH-secreting-adenomas is indefinite and no definite role for various oncogenes has been demonstrated (70). Based on the Clarke et al. study, these tumors are often delayed in diagnosis, are frequently macroadenomas and plurihormonal in terms of their pathological characteristics, have a heterogeneous clinical picture, and are difficult to treat (71). Sometimes mixed pituitary tumors co-secrete TSH, growth hormone and prolactin (70).

### 5.1 Symptoms

Because of the long standing duration of the disease, patients present mild or moderate signs of hyperthyroidism and can rarely be asymptomatic (68, 72, 73). In addition, mass effects of the pituitary tumor such as loss of vision and visual field defects may be occurred (70, 73). Moreover, hyperthyroid features can be eclipsed by those of acromegaly in patients with mixed TSH/GH adenomas, thus emphasizing the importance of systematic measurement of TSH and free thyroxin (FT4) in patients with pituitary tumor (74).

### 5.2 Epidemiology

TSH secreting tumors account for 0.9 to 2.8% percent of all pituitary adenomas. The diagnosis of these tumors has been increasing in the past 20 years (69). Most patients have macroadenomas, and microadenomas are exceptional (75).

### 5.3 Diagnosis

Hormonal evaluation shows increased free thyroid hormone concentration with detectable, normal or increased serum TSH level, raising the differential diagnosis of pituitary resistance to thyroid hormone (72). Ultrasensitive TSH assays allow a clear distinction between patients with suppressed and those with non-suppressed circulating TSH concentrations, i.e. between patients with primary hyperthyroidism (Graves' disease or toxic nodular goiter) and those with central hyperthyroidism (TSH-secreting adenomas or pituitary resistance to thyroid hormone action) (73). The MRI discloses the pituitary adenoma (72). A (99 m) Tc-octreotide scan can be a useful tool for confirming diagnosis of TSH-secreting adenoma (76).

### 5.4 Management

Therapy of TSH-secreting adenomas can be accomplished by surgery, radiation therapy, and medical treatment with somatostatin analogs or dopamine agonists (70).

The major aim is to remove the pituitary tumor and restore euthyroidism. Thus, the first therapeutic approach to TSH-secreting pituitary microadenomas should be the transsphenoidal or subfrontal adenomectomy, the choice of the route depending on the tumor volume and its suprasellar extension. This may be complex because of the occasional marked fibrosis of these tumors, possibly related to high expression of basic fibroblast growth factor (68, 77). In patients with macroadenomas or invasive pituitary tumors, long-acting somatostatin analogs may be an effective therapeutic measure to decrease TSH and thyroid hormone secretion (72, 78). Octreotide can control central hyperthyroidism, induce tumor shrinkage, and it can be a satisfactory method of preoperative preparation for TSH-secreting adenoma (73, 76). Aberrant expression of TRβ4 (a novel thyroid hormone receptor β isoform) could possibly contribute to the aberrant secretion of TSH in a TSH-secreting adenoma (79).

### 5.5 Outcome

In the past, about one third of the patients were diagnosed as having a primary hyperthyroidism (Graves' disease) and thus mistakenly were treated with thyroid ablation (thyroidectomy and/or radioiodine) (73).

The increasing frequency and early diagnosis of TSH secreting pituitary adenoma may be explained by ultrasensitive methods now used for TSH measurement and progress in pituitary imaging, mainly with MRI. This change in the presentation and the state of disease at diagnosis and the excellent response to somatostatins has improved the prognosis for this uncommon disease (70, 80).

### 5.6 Complications

Failure to recognize the presence of a TSH-secreting adenoma may result in dramatic consequences, such as improper thyroid ablation that may cause the pituitary tumor volume to further expand (73).

## 6. LH and FSH secreting PA

Recent studies have found that a high proportion of clinically non-functioning pituitary adenomas are largely gonadotrope-derived, i.e. produce and secrete low levels of intact follicle-stimulating hormone (FSH), luteinizing hormone (LH) or only biologically inert alpha- or beta-subunits of these hormones (81, 82).

### 6.1 Symptoms

Gonadotroph adenomas are not typically associated with a clinical syndrome (2). They are almost always discovered in patients presenting with mass effect, including visual field loss and headache, hypogonadism, and hypopituitarism (81). Anterior pituitary insufficiency is much more frequent than gonadal hyperstimulation such as ovarian hyperstimulation (83), testicular enlargement (82), and precocious puberty (81, 84).

### 6.2 Epidemiology

Advances in immunocytochemistry, electron microscopy, cell culture, and molecular techniques have demonstrated that 80 to 90% of the clinically nonfunctioning pituitary adenomas are gonadotrope-derived and recently recognized as gonadotropinomas, which account for as many as 40 to 50% of all pituitary macroadenomas (81, 84). Gonadotropinomas have been reported with increasing frequency in middle-aged men, but they are less frequently recognized in women. This could be the result of greater difficulty in diagnosis due to the normal increase in serum gonadotropins in postmenopausal women (85).

### 6.3 Diagnosis

Both clinical and hormonal characteristics of gonadotropinomas usually make them readily distinguishable from pituitary enlargement due to long-standing primary hypogonadism (86). A careful analysis of hormone assay results show that baseline concentrations of gonadotrophin or their free sub-units are elevated in 30 to 50% of the cases. The GnRH test is positive in 75 to 100% of the cases (84). The majority of the cases can be recognized, even in postmenopausal women, by the serum LH beta responses to TRH, and some can be recognized by the responses of serum FSH and LH (87, 88).

### 6.4 Management

Most gonadotropinomas are now first treated by transsphenoidal surgery, to make an attempt to restore vision as quickly as possible, and then by radiation therapy to prevent the regrowth of any remaining adenomatous tissue. Radiosurgery using gamma knife, the linear accelerator, or proton beam therapy showed promising results, especially for controlling residual or recurrent tumors (63, 81). Medical therapy for a gonadotrope adenoma with a somatostatin analogs, dopamine agonists, or GnRH agonists and antagonists has limited utility but is employed in patients who are unable to undergo surgery. They may delay or prevent additional tumor growth (64, 84, 89, 90). Experimental therapy with intraoperative local chemotherapy or potential gene therapy requires further investigation (81).

### 6.5 Outcome & Complications

Long-term outcomes and complications of gonadotropinomas are similar to those of non-functioning pituitary adenomas.

## 7. Acknowledgements

The authors thank Mrs. Bita Pourmand for her edit of the chapter.

## 8. References

[1] McDowell B, Wallace R, Carnahan R, Chrischilles E, Lynch C, Schlechte J. Demographic differences in incidence for pituitary adenoma. Pituitary. 2011;14(1):23-30.

[2] Greenberg MS. Handbook of Neurosurgery. 7 ed. New York: Thieme Medical Pub; 2010.

[3] Ebersold MJ, Quast LM, Laws ER, Jr., Scheithauer B, Randall RV. Long-term results in transsphenoidal removal of nonfunctioning pituitary adenomas. J Neurosurg. 1986 May;64(5):713-9.

[4] Verhelst J, Abs R. Hyperprolactinemia: pathophysiology and management. Treat Endocrinol. 2003;2(1):23-32.
[5] Anonymous. Pituitary Adenoma (Tumor).2011; http://neurosurgery.ucla.edu [cited 2011 8/8/2011]
[6] Mah PM, Webster J. Hyperprolactinemia: etiology, diagnosis, and management. Semin Reprod Med. 2002;20(4):365-74.
[7] Hoffman AR, Melmed S, Schlechte J. Patient guide to hyperprolactinemia diagnosis and treatment. J Clin Endocrinol Metab. 2011;96(2):35A-6A.
[8] Mancini T, Casanueva FF, Giustina A. Hyperprolactinemia and prolactinomas. Endocrinol Metab Clin North Am. 2008;37(1):67-99, viii.
[9] Coppola A, Cuomo MA. Prolactinoma in the male. Physiopathological, clinical, and therapeutic features. Minerva Endocrinol. 1998;23(1):7-16. [Italian]
[10] Colao A, Lombardi G. Growth hormone and prolactin excess. Lancet. 1998;352:1455-61.
[11] Gillam MP, Molitch ME, Lombardi G, Colao A. Advances in the treatment of prolactinomas. Endocr Rev. 2006;27(5):485-534.
[12] Colao A, Savastano S. Medical treatment of prolactinomas. Nat Rev Endocrinol. 2011;7(5):267-78.
[13] Colao A. Pituitary tumours: the prolactinoma. Best Pract Res Clin Endocrinol Metab. 2009 Oct;23(5):575-96.
[14] Biller BM. Diagnostic evaluation of hyperprolactinemia. J Reprod Med. 1999;44(12 Suppl):1095-9.
[15] Cunnah D, Besser M. Management of prolactinomas. Clin Endocrinol (Oxf). 1991;34(3):231-5.
[16] Colao A, Di Sarno A, Guerra E, De Leo M, Mentone A, Lombardi G. Drug insight: Cabergoline and bromocriptine in the treatment of hyperprolactinemia in men and women. Nat Clin Pract Endocrinol Metab. 2006;2(4):200-10.
[17] Crosignani PG. Current treatment issues in female hyperprolactinaemia. Eur J Obstet Gynecol Reprod Biol. 2006;125(2):152-64.
[18] Dekkers OM, Lagro J, Burman P, Jorgensen JO, Romijn JA, Pereira AM. Recurrence of hyperprolactinemia after withdrawal of dopamine agonists: systematic review and meta-analysis. J Clin Endocrinol Metab. 2010;95(1):43-51.
[19] Barlier A, Jaquet P. Quinagolide--a valuable treatment option for hyperprolactinaemia. Eur J Endocrinol. 2006;154(2):187-95.
[20] Orrego JJ, Chandler WF, Barkan AL. Pergolide as primary therapy for macroprolactinomas. Pituitary. 2000;3(4):251-6.
[21] Ono M, Miki N, Amano K, Kawamata T, Seki T, Makino R, et al. Individualized high-dose cabergoline therapy for hyperprolactinemic infertility in women with micro- and macroprolactinomas. J Clin Endocrinol Metab. 2010;95(6):2672-9.
[22] Jan M, Dufour H, Brue T, Jaquet P. Prolactinoma surgery. Ann Endocrinol (Paris). 2007;68(2-3):118-9.
[23] Sasaki R, Murakami M, Okamoto Y, Kono K, Yoden E, Nakajima T, et al. The efficacy of conventional radiation therapy in the management of pituitary adenoma. International Journal of Radiation Oncology, Biology, Physics. 2000;47(5):1337-45.
[24] Akabane A, Yamada S, Jokura H. Gamma knife radiosurgery for pituitary adenomas. Endocrine. 2005;28(1):87-91.

[25] Schlechte JA. Long-Term Management of Prolactinomas. Journal of Clinical Endocrinology & Metabolism. 2007;92(8):2861-5.
[26] Zhen JR, Yu Q, Zhang YH, Ma WB, Lin SQ. Cost-effectiveness analysis of two therapeutic methods for prolactinoma. Zhonghua Fu Chan Ke Za Zhi. 2008;43(4):257-61. [Chinese]
[27] Kars M, Pereira AM, Smit JW, Romijn JA. Long-term outcome of patients with macroprolactinomas initially treated with dopamine agonists. European Journal of Internal Medicine. 2009;20(4):387-93.
[28] Jane JA, Jr., Laws ER, Jr. The surgical management of pituitary adenomas in a series of 3,093 patients. J Am Coll Surg. 2001;193(6):651-9.
[29] Brada M, Ashley S, Ford D, Traish D, Burchell L, Rajan B. Cerebrovascular mortality in patients with pituitary adenoma. Clin Endocrinol (Oxf). 2002;57(6):713-7.
[30] Erem C, Kocak M, Nuhoglu I, Yilmaz M, Ucuncu O. Blood coagulation, fibrinolysis and lipid profile in patients with prolactinoma. Clin Endocrinol (Oxf). 2010;73(4):502-7.
[31] Hurtado Amador R, Ayala AR, Hernandez Marin I. [The impact of prolactinoma in human reproduction]. Ginecol Obstet Mex. 2004;72(1):3-9.
[32] Suzuki K, Hattori Y, Aoki C, Nakano A, Tomizawa A, Kase H, et al. An ACTH-secreting pituitary adenoma within the sphenoid sinus. Intern Med. 2010;49(8):763-6.
[33] Nieman LK, Biller BMK, Findling JW, Newell-Price J, Savage MO, Stewart PM, et al. The Diagnosis of Cushing's Syndrome: An Endocrine Society Clinical Practice Guideline. Journal of Clinical Endocrinology & Metabolism. 2008, 2008;93(5):1526-40.
[34] Newell-Price J, Bertagna X, Grossman AB, Nieman LK. Cushing's syndrome. The Lancet. 2006;367(9522):1605-17.
[35] Findling JW, Raff H. Cushing's Syndrome: Important Issues in Diagnosis and Management. Journal of Clinical Endocrinology & Metabolism. 2006, 2006;91(10):3746-53.
[36] Tauchmanovà L, Pivonello R, Di Somma C, Rossi R, De Martino MC, Camera L, et al. Bone Demineralization and Vertebral Fractures in Endogenous Cortisol Excess: Role of Disease Etiology and Gonadal Status. Journal of Clinical Endocrinology & Metabolism. 2006;91(5):1779-84.
[37] Mancini T, Kola B, Mantero F, Boscaro M, Arnaldi G. High cardiovascular risk in patients with Cushing's syndrome according to 1999 WHO/ISH guidelines. Clinical Endocrinology. 2004;61(6):768-77.
[38] Muiesan ML, Lupia M, Salvetti M, Grigoletto C, Sonino N, Boscaro M, et al. Left ventricular structural and functional characteristics in Cushing's syndrome. Journal of the American College of Cardiology. 2003;41(12):2275-9.
[39] Arnaldi G, Angeli A, Atkinson AB, Bertagna X, Cavagnini F, Chrousos GP, et al. Diagnosis and Complications of Cushing's Syndrome: A Consensus Statement. Journal of Clinical Endocrinology & Metabolism. 2003;88(12):5593-602.
[40] Sonino N, Bonnini S, Fallo F, Boscaro M, Fava GA. Personality characteristics and quality of life in patients treated for Cushing's syndrome. Clinical Endocrinology. 2006;64(3):314-8.
[41] Forget H, Lacroix A, Cohen H. Persistent cognitive impairment following surgical treatment of Cushing's syndrome. Psychoneuroendocrinology. 2002;27(3):367-83.

[42] Banasiak MJ, Malek AR. Nelson syndrome: comprehensive review of pathophysiology, diagnosis, and management. Neurosurg Focus. 2007;23(3):E13.
[43] Santos S, Santos E, Gaztambide S, Salvador J. Diagnóstico y diagnóstico diferencial del síndrome de Cushing. Endocrinología y Nutrición. 2009;56(2):71-84.
[44] Elamin MB, Murad MH, Mullan R, Erickson D, Harris K, Nadeem S, et al. Accuracy of Diagnostic Tests for Cushing's Syndrome: A Systematic Review and Metaanalyses. Journal of Clinical Endocrinology & Metabolism. 2008 May 1, 2008;93(5):1553-62.
[45] Beauregard C, Dickstein G, Lacroix A. Classic and Recent Etiologies of Cushing's Syndrome: Diagnosis and Therapy. Treatments in Endocrinology. 2002;1(2):79-94.
[46] Bertagna X, Guignat L, Groussin L, Bertherat J. Cushing's disease. Best Practice & Research Clinical Endocrinology & Metabolism. 2009;23(5):607-23.
[47] Jagannathan J, Smith R, DeVroom HL, Vortmeyer AO, Stratakis CA, Nieman LK, et al. Outcome of using the histological pseudocapsule as a surgical capsule in Cushing disease. J Neurosurg. 2009;111(3):531-9.
[48] Kobayashi T, Kida Y, Mori Y. Gamma knife radiosurgery in the treatment of Cushing disease: long-term results. J Neurosurg. 2002;97(5 Suppl):422-8.
[49] Castinetti F, Nagai M, Dufour H, Kuhn J-M, Morange I, Jaquet P, et al. Gamma knife radiosurgery is a successful adjunctive treatment in Cushing's disease. European Journal of Endocrinology. 2007;156(1):91-8.
[50] Atkinson AB, Kennedy A, Wiggam MI, McCance DR, Sheridan B. Long-term remission rates after pituitary surgery for Cushing's disease: the need for long-term surveillance. Clin Endocrinol (Oxf). 2005;63(5):549-59.
[51] Ohmori N, Nomura K, Ohmori K, Kato Y, Itoh T, Takano K. Osteoporosis is more prevalent in adrenal than in pituitary Cushing's syndrome. Endocr J. 2003;50(1):1-7.
[52] Bourdeau I, Bard C, Noël B, Leclerc I, Cordeau M-P, Bélair M, et al. Loss of Brain Volume in Endogenous Cushing's Syndrome and Its Reversibility after Correction of Hypercortisolism. Journal of Clinical Endocrinology & Metabolism. 2002;87(5):1949-54.
[53] van Aken MO, Pereira AM, Biermasz NR, van Thiel SW, Hoftijzer HC, Smit JWA, et al. Quality of Life in Patients after Long-Term Biochemical Cure of Cushing's Disease. Journal of Clinical Endocrinology & Metabolism. 2005;90(6):3279-86.
[54] Feelders RA, Hofland LJ, van Aken MO, Neggers SJ, Lamberts SWJ, de Herder WW, et al. Medical Therapy of Acromegaly: Efficacy and Safety of Somatostatin Analogues. Drugs. 2009;69(16):2207-26
[55] Chanson P, Salenave S, Kamenicky P, Cazabat L, Young J. Acromegaly. Best Practice & Research Clinical Endocrinology & Metabolism. 2009;23(5):555-74.
[56] Melmed S. Acromegaly pathogenesis and treatment. J Clin Invest. 2009;119(11):3189-202.
[57] Chanson P, Salenave S. Acromegaly. Orphanet J Rare Dis. 2008;3:17.
[58] Scacchi M, Cavagnini F. Acromegaly. Pituitary. 2006;9(4):297-303.
[59] Chanson P. [Acromegaly]. Presse Med. 2009;38(1):92-102.
[60] Giustina A, Barkan A, Casanueva FF, Cavagnini F, Frohman L, Ho K, et al. Criteria for Cure of Acromegaly: A Consensus Statement. Journal of Clinical Endocrinology & Metabolism. 2000;85(2):526-9.
[61] Trainer PJ. Acromegaly—Consensus, What Consensus? Journal of Clinical Endocrinology & Metabolism. 2002;87(8):3534-6.

[62] Giustina A, Casanueva FF, Cavagnini F, Chanson P, Clemmons D, Frohman LA, et al. Diagnosis and treatment of acromegaly complications. J Endocrinol Invest. 2003;26(12):1242-7.

[63] Chanson P, Salenave S. Diagnosis and treatment of pituitary adenomas. Minerva Endocrinol. 2004;29(4):241-75.

[64] Vance ML. Medical treatment of functional pituitary tumors. Neurosurg Clin N Am. 2003;14(1):81-7.

[65] Maiza JC, Vezzosi D, Matta M, Donadille F, Loubes-Lacroix F, Cournot M, et al. Long-term (up to 18 years) effects on GH/IGF-1 hypersecretion and tumour size of primary somatostatin analogue (SSTa) therapy in patients with GH-secreting pituitary adenoma responsive to SSTa. Clin Endocrinol (Oxf). 2007;67(2):282-9.

[66] Clemmons DR, Chihara K, Freda PU, Ho KKY, Klibanski A, Melmed S, et al. Optimizing Control of Acromegaly: Integrating a Growth Hormone Receptor Antagonist into the Treatment Algorithm. Journal of Clinical Endocrinology & Metabolism. 2003;88(10):4759-67.

[67] Colao A, Ferone D, Marzullo P, Lombardi G. Systemic Complications of Acromegaly: Epidemiology, Pathogenesis, and Management. Endocrine Reviews. 2004;25(1):102-52.

[68] Jha S, Kumar S. TSH secreting pituitary adenoma. J Assoc Physicians India. 2009;57:537-9.

[69] Zielinski G, Podgorski JK, Warczynska A, Koziarski A, Zgliczynski W. Thyrotropin--TSH secreting pituitary tumor. Przegl Lek. 2002;59(12):1018-23. [Polish]

[70] Losa M, Fortunato M, Molteni L, Peretti E, Mortini P. Thyrotropin-secreting pituitary adenomas: biological and molecular features, diagnosis and therapy. Minerva Endocrinol. 2008;33(4):329-40.

[71] Clarke MJ, Erickson D, Castro MR, Atkinson JL. Thyroid-stimulating hormone pituitary adenomas. J Neurosurg. 2008;109(1):17-22.

[72] Caron P. Thyrotropin-secreting pituitary adenomas. Presse Med. 2009;38(1):107-11. [French]

[73] Beck-Peccoz P, Persani L. Medical Management of Thyrotropin-Secreting Pituitary Adenomas. Pituitary. 2002;5(2):83-8.

[74] Losa M, Giovanelli M, Persani L, Mortini P, Faglia G, Beck-Peccoz P. Criteria of cure and follow-up of central hyperthyroidism due to thyrotropin-secreting pituitary adenomas. J Clin Endocrinol Metab. 1996;81(8):3084-90.

[75] Calvo Romero JM, Morales Perez F, Alvarez Barreiro JA, Diaz Perez de Madrid J. Thyrotropin-producing hypophyseal adenomas. Rev Clin Esp. 1999;199(5):285-7. [Spanish]

[76] Chen S, Li M, Lian XL, Zeng ZP, Dai WX, Li F, et al. Octreotide in the diagnosis and treatment of pituitary thyrotropin-secreting adenoma. Zhonghua Nei Ke Za Zhi. 2006;45(11):910-3. [Chinese]

[77] Ezzat S, Horvath E, Kovacs K, Smyth HS, Singer W, Asa SL. Basic Fibroblast Growth Factor Expression by Two Prolactin and Thyrotropin-Producing Pituitary Adenomas. Endocr Pathol. 1995;6(2):125-34.

[78] Yoenem A, Cakyr B, Azal O, Corakcy A, Kutlu M, Oezata M. Effect of octreotide acetate on thyrotropin-secreting adenoma: report of two cases and review of the literature. Endocr Regul. 1999;33(4):169-74.

[79] Tagami T, Usui T, Shimatsu A, Beniko M, Yamamoto H, Moriyama K, et al. Aberrant expression of thyroid hormone receptor beta isoform may cause inappropriate secretion of TSH in a TSH-secreting pituitary adenoma. J Clin Endocrinol Metab. 2011;96(6):E948-52.

[80] Latrech H, Rousseau A, Le Marois E, Billaud L, Bertagna X, Azzoug S, et al. Présentation et pronostic des adénomes thyréotropes : à propos de trois observations. La Revue de Médecine Interne. 2010;31(12):858-62.

[81] Chaidarun SS, Klibanski A. Gonadotropinomas. Semin Reprod Med. 2002;20(4):339-48.

[82] Dahlqvist P, Koskinen L-O, Brännström T, Hägg E. Testicular enlargement in a patient with a FSH-secreting pituitary adenoma. Endocrine. 2010;37(2):289-93.

[83] Cooper O, Geller JL, Melmed S. Ovarian hyperstimulation syndrome caused by an FSH-secreting pituitary adenoma. Nat Clin Pract Endocrinol Metab. 2008;4(4):234-8.

[84] Chanson P. [Gonadotroph pituitary adenomas]. Ann Endocrinol (Paris). 2000;61(3):258-68.

[85] Hattori N, Ishihara T, Moridera K, Ikekubo K, Hino M, Saiki Y, et al. LH- and FSH-secreting pituitary adenoma in a postmenopausal woman. Endocrinol Jpn. 1991;38(4):393-6.

[86] Snyder PJ. Gonadotroph cell adenomas of the pituitary. Endocr Rev. 1985;6(4):552-63.

[87] Daneshdoost L, Gennarelli TA, Bashey HM, Savino PJ, Sergott RC, Bosley TM, et al. Recognition of gonadotroph adenomas in women. N Engl J Med. 1991;324(9):589-94.

[88] Gruszka A, Kunert-Radek J, Pawlikowski M. Serum alpha-subunit elevation after TRH administration: a valuable test in presurgical diagnosis of gonadotropinoma? Endokrynol Pol. 2005;56(1):14-8.

[89] Berezin M, Olchovsky D, Pines A, Tadmor R, Lunenfeld B. Reduction of follicle-stimulating hormone (FSH) secretion in FSH-producing pituitary adenoma by bromocriptine. J Clin Endocrinol Metab. 1984;59(6):1220-3.

[90] Chanson P, Brochier S. Non-functioning pituitary adenomas. J Endocrinol Invest. 2005;28(11 Suppl International):93-9.

# 4

# Pituitary Adenomas – Clinico-Pathological, Immunohistochemical and Ultrastructural Study

Alma Ortiz-Plata, Martha L. Tena-Suck, Iván Pérez-Neri, Daniel Rembao-Bojórquez and Angeles Fernández
*National Institute of Neurology and Neurosurgery*
*México City*
*México*

## 1. Introduction

Pituitary adenomas (PA) constitute about 10% of intracranial neoplasm. Most of them have its origin in adenohypophysis (Cury et al., 2009; Rosai, 1989). They occur most often in adults between the ages of 30 and 60 years, and may have slightly higher incidence in females in early life (20-45 years) and in males in later life (35-60 years) (Davis et al., 2001; McDowell et al., 2011). The majority of pituitary adenomas have a sporadic origin; familial cases represent 5% of all pituitary tumors (Vandeva et al., 2010; Tichomirowa et al., 2009). Couldwell and Cannon (2010) report strong evidence of genetic contribution for predisposition to symptomatic pituitary tumors.

Pituitary adenomas clinically manifest by signs of hypopituitarism, this is caused by the compression of the gland by the tumor which may affect fertility, the compression of other adjacent structures may cause headache and if the optic chiasm is affected visual alterations; secretion of one or more specific hormones can take place (Galland & Chanson, 2009; Melmed, 2010). However, up to 30% of adenomas do not secrete hormones (Cury et al., 2009; Martinez, 1986; Moreno, 2005).

Pituitary adenomas have been classified as: microadenomas (<10mm diameter) and macroadenomas (> 10 mm diameter), according to its size assessed by tomography and magnetic resonance; staining affinity (acidophilic, chromophobic or basophilic); hormonal activity or secretion of growth hormone (GH), prolactin (PRL), thyroid stimulating hormone(TSH), adrenocorticotrophin hormone (ACTH), follicle stimulating hormone (FSH), and luteinizing hormone (LH); and ultrastructural characteristics (Galland & Chanson, 2009; Nosé, 2011). Hardy (1973) classified pituitary adenomas in four grades according to its size and local invasion degree:

Grade I: Microadenomas, measuring less than 10mm in diameter, they minimally alter the radiographic appearance of the sella.
Grade II: Macroadenomas are bigger than 10mm in diameter, they enlarge the sella or exhibit suprasellar expansion, but not cause destruction.
Grade III: Invasive adenomas, locally eroded the sella, and show suprasellar outgrowth.
Grade IV: Strongly invasive adenomas, that destroys adjacent bony structures and with suprasellar outgrowth, including bone, hypothalamus, and the cavernous sinus.

This classification remains valid using computed tomography scanning and magnetic resonance imaging.

Histologically pituitary adenomas are dense cellular tumors, composed by cells with solid nuclei, rounded and uniform. These cells can be arranged in big groups (diffused pattern), around sinusoidal vessels (sinusoidal pattern), or covering connective-vascular axes (papillary pattern). In all PA types, atypia and mitotic cells are rare. Despite the histologically benign aspect, pituitary adenomas may have an invasive behavior (Chang, 2010; Lau, et al., 2010; Li-Ng, 2008; Melmed, 2010; Scheithauer, 1986; Zada et al., 2011;). This factor is not necessarily indicative of malignancy, because tumor growth is slow and metastases are rare. The histological aspect is not different from the rare carcinoma cases (Colao et al., 2010; Crocker, 1978; Kaltsas et al., 2005; Schteithauer et al., 2005; Tena-Suck et al., 2006;).

In most patients the pathologist cannot provide information about the PA behavior, if will be aggressive based on the histological appearance of adenomas, this is because tumors with variations in the size, shape and nuclear density and the presence of bi-or multinucleated cells do not necessarily had a poor prognosis.

The functional classification of pituitary adenomas based on its hormonal activity, assessed by immunohistochemistry technique, and associated with the transmission electron microscopy analysis, has allowed the characterization of neoplastic cells in detail and proposes the classification of the adenomas in 14 different types, this allows a better correlation with the clinical manifestations that the old classification of chromophobe, acidophilic and basophilic pituitary adenomas (Horvath & Kovacs, 1992; Horvath, 1994; Kovacs & Horvath, 1986).

The aim of this investigation is to present a review of different cases of pituitary adenomas studied in the Laboratory of Experimental Neuropathology of National Institute of Neurology and Neurosurgery, correlating the local invasion degree, clinical manifestations, histological aspects, immunohistochemical and ultrastructural features, with the biological behavior, especially with the invasive potential.

## 2. Methods

One hundred and twenty two cases of pituitary adenomas were studied. They were classified by their local invasion degree according with Hardy classification (Hardy, 1973), endocrine symptoms (clinically functioning and clinically non functioning pituitary adenomas) and by their hormonal secretion, assessed by immunohistochemistry. The evolution of the disease at the time of diagnosis, tumor regrowth, bromocriptine treatment, and time of outcome of the patients, were evaluated to analyze the PA biological behavior.

### 2.1 Histopathological analysis

The biopsies were divided in two parts; the first one was fixed in phosphate-buffer saline (PBS)-formalin solution, alcohol dehydrated and paraffin-embedded. Five µm sections were stained with hematoxilyn-eosin and Masson's trichrome (Prophet & Arrington, 1992) for PA treated with bomocriptine. In each hematoxylin-eosin stained section was analyzed nuclear pleomorphism and mitosis figures.

### 2.2 Immunohistochemistry

In other sections, immunohistochemistry (Bratthauer et al., 1994) was performed. Slides of each case were deparaffinized, rehydrated, and rinsed in PBS. Later on, endogenous peroxidase was blocked with 0.25 % $H_2O_2$/distilled water for 15 min., and blocking with 3% BSA in PBS (Albumin, Bovine, Sigma-AldrichCo. St. Louis USA). The slides were incubated for 1 h in ready to use monoclonal antibodies of pituitary hormones: prolactin, growth hormone (GH), luteinizing hormone (LH), follicle-stimulating hormone (FSH), thyroid stimulating hormone (TSH) (BioGenex, San Ramón, CA) and adrenocorticotropic hormone (ACTH, DAKO, Carpinteria, Ca, at a 1;100 dilution). Normal postmortem pituitaries were used as positive controls for pituitary hormones. To assess the proliferative index of pituitary adenomas Ki-67 antibody was used (Santa Cruz Biotechnology, inc. Santa Cruz CA. USA at 1:100 dilution). After that the sections were washed, and incubated for 30 min. with the secondary antibody (biotinylated anti-Ig, BioGenex, San Ramón, CA). After washing in PBS the sections were incubated for 30 min with peroxidase-conjugated streptavidina complex (BioGenex, San Ramón, CA). The reaction was developed with diaminobenzidine (DAB) using a Dako kit detection system (Dako enVision System Peroxidase. Dako Carpinteria, CA) according to manufacturer's instructions and the sections were hematoxylin counterstained. The immunodetection was analyzed under a wide-field microscope Olympus H2 (Tokyo, Japan). The immunoreactivity to different hormones in tumor cells were estimated as positive or negative, and the Ki-67 labeled index (LI) was assessed by counting the percentage of number of positive / nuclear cells in five 40x fields. Statistics analysis were done to associate Ki-67 labeling index (LI), disease evolution time, and outcome, in functional PA and in non-functional PA, hormone secretion, invasion degree, and tumor regrowth.

### 2.3 Ultrastructural analysis

The second part of biopsy was processed for its use in electron microscopy to assess the fine structure of PA. The tissues were fixed in 2.5% glutaraldehyde in 0.1 M phosphate-buffer-saline (PBS pH 7.4) and postfixed in 1% tetroxide osmium in the same buffer, dehydrated in alcohol, and embedded in Epon. One-micron thick sections were stained with toluidine blue and examined by light microscopy. Ultrathin sections at the silver/grey area of the spectrum of interference colors were stained with uranyl acetate and lead citrate and examined under Zeiss EM 10 transmission electron microscopy.

### 2.4 Statistical analysis

Statistical analysis was performed by using the SPSS 13.0 software. ANOVA test and $X^2$, Kurskal-Wallis were used to evaluate differences and association respectively, among evolution time and follow up with grades of invasion. Bivariate analysis was accomplished by means of Fisher's exact test for association among functional and non-functional PA, or hormonal immunodetection with recurrences. U Mann-Whitney's test was used to assess evolution time and follow up differences among functioning and non-functioning PA. To evaluate differences in Ki-67-LI detection among invasion grades, $X^2$ Kurskal-Wallis test was done; among functioning and non-functioning PA with recurrences U Mann-Whitney's test was used; and the association of Ki-67-LI detection with hormonal immunodetection, U Mann-Whitney's test was accomplished. P value less than .05 were considered significant.

## 3. Results

One hundred and twenty two pituitary adenomas were studied between 1988 and 1992. They were organized according to their characteristics, by means of transsphenoidal or transcranial-frontal technique, and the tumors were removed in 60 to 100%. Tumors mainly affected young adult population with a mean age of 41.4 yr. Sixty five (53.3%) were male, mean age of 43.6±14.8 yr (range, 17-71 yr) and 57 (46.7%) were female, mean age of 39.3±14.4 yr (range, 13-75 yr). Twelve patients were under 20 yr (9.8%). Six males with mean age of 18.8 ± 2.4 yr, and 6 females with mean age of 16.1 ± 2.5 yr. Clinically they were 11 functioning PA and 1 non-functioning PA (Table 1).

| Grade | Gender | Age (yr) | Evolution Time (yr) | F | NF | Symptoms | IHQ |
|---|---|---|---|---|---|---|---|
| II | M | 17 | 1 | X | | Hypogonadism | Prl |
| II | M | 20 | 2 | X | | VA Ha Ac | GH |
| II | F | 23 | 4 | X | | VA Ha Am-Gal | Prl-TSH |
| II | M | 24 | 6 | X | | Cush | Neg |
| II | M | 18 | 4 | | X | VA Ha | Prl |
| III | F | 14 | 2 | X | | VA Am | Prl |
| III | M | 20 | 8 | X | | Gal-Am Gig | Prl-GH |
| III | F | 23 | 8 | X | | VA Ha Am-Gal | Prl-ACTH |
| IV | F | 18 | 4 | X | | VA Ha Am | Prl |
| IV | F | 18 | 4 | X | | VA Ha Am-Gal | Neg |
| IV | F | 13 | 2 | X | | VA Am | Prl |
| IV | M | 20 | 2 | X | | VA Ac | Prl-GH |

F= functioning pituitary adenoma; NF= non-functioning pituitary adenoma; VA= visual alterations; Ha= headache; Am= amenorrhea; Gal= Galactorrhea; Gig= gigantism; Ac= acromegaly; IHQ= immunohistochemical detection.

Table 1. Pituitary adenomas in young cases under 20 years old at the onset of symptoms. The age column is the age at diagnosis.

Twenty two cases (18%) were classified as I and II invasion grades tumors, and 66 cases (54.1%) were in extensive invasion phase (IV grade). The disease evolution time before the first surgery was 2.9±2.3 yr (range, 2 months to 10 years). Of the 122 patients thirty eight patients continued to attend their review appointments (31%). The average follow up time of the patients was 11±7.4 yr (range, 1-27 yr); from 1 to 5 yr, and from 15 to 20 yr, were the most frequent. Only one patient (0.8%) was considered healthy; four deaths have been reported. The remaining patients stopped coming to the Institute to control appointments. Thirty nine (31.9%) cases out of the 122 had recurrence; 23 (58.9%) belong to grade IV PA. In grade III and IV, two patients with recurrences were observed (Table 2).

| Grade | Cases n | Gender Female n(%) | Mean Age F/M | Evolution Time Years (mean) | Follow up time Years (range) | Recurrences | | |
|---|---|---|---|---|---|---|---|---|
| | | | | | | Cases n (%) | 1 | 2 |
| I | 2 | 1 (50) | 33/31 | 1.5 | 1 | 0 | | |
| II | 20 | 4 (20%) | 39/45 | 2.1 | 10.6 (1m-20yr) | 6 (15.3%) | 6 | |
| III | 34 | 23 (67%) | 40/34 | 3.4 | 12.1 (2-20) | 10 (25.6%) | 7 | 3 |
| IV | 66 | 29 (44%) | 39/44 | 3 | 10.3 (1-27) | 23 (58.9%) | 21 | 2 |

Table 2. Pituitary adenomas classification by grades of invasion according to Hardy (1973). Disease evolution time, follow up time, and recurrences in each grade are shown.
F= females; M= males; m= month.

### 3.1 Immunohistochemistry

Prolactin was the most frequent hormone detected by immunohistochemistry (54 cases, 44.2%) (Table 3). Prolactin hormone expression was found in combination with others hormones: 10 were in combination with GH (8.1%), 4 (3.2%) with TSH; 3 (2.4%) with ACTH, and 1 (0.81%) with LH. Fifteen (12.3%) cases were positive for gonadotroph hormones, 5 (4%) for growth hormone, 2 (1.6%) for ACTH, 1 (0.82%) for TSH, 1 (0.82%) multihormonal (HC-FSH-TSH), and 26 (21.3%) cases were negative for all hormones (Fig. 1).

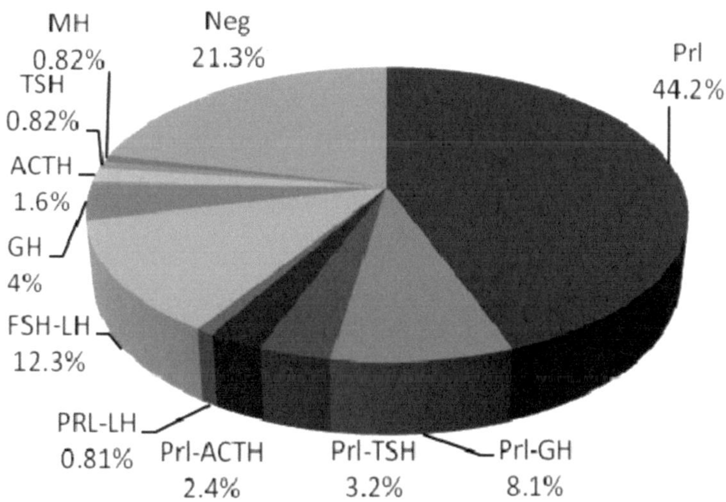


Fig. 1. Pituitary adenoma classification according to their hormonal content assessed by immunohistochemistry.
Prolactin hormone expression was the most frequent detected. Prl= prolactin hormone; GH= Growth hormone; TSH= Thyroid stimulating hormone; ACTH= adrenocorticotropin hormone; LH= luteinizing hormone; FSH= follicle stimulating hormone; MH= multihormonal; Neg= negative.

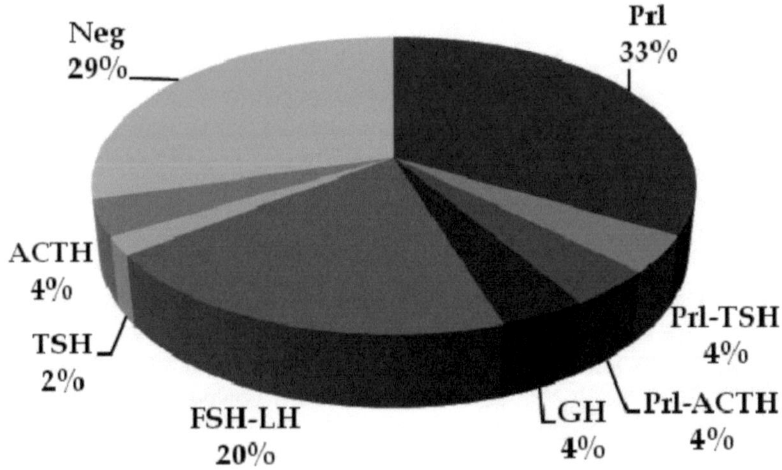


Fig. 2. Classification of non-functioning pituitary adenomas.
Immunohistochemical detection of hormonal expression in non-functioning pituitary adenomas. Prl= prolactin hormone; GH= Growth hormone; TSH= Thyroid stimulating hormone; ACTH= adrenocorticotropin hormone; LH= luteinizing hormone; FSH= follicle stimulating hormone; Neg= negative.

There were 51 (41.8%) non-functioning PA, 17 (33%) were Prl positive by immunohistochemistry, 15 (29%) were negative, and 10 (19.6%) were positive for gonadotrophic hormones (Fig. 2).

Non-functioning PA presented visual alterations and headache as clinical manifestations. There was 58.2% of clinically functioning pituitary adenomas. The most frequent clinical manifestations were: amenorrhea, galactorrhea, and libido diminished. Acromegaly was found in GH positive pituitary adenomas and one patient with gigantism was found (Table 1). Ki-67-LI was high in IV grade tumors (Table 3, Fig. 3).

| Grade | Cases # | F | NF | Prl # (%) | Ki-67-LI Median (range) |
|---|---|---|---|---|---|
| I | 2 | 2 | - | 2 (100) | ND |
| II | 20 | 10 | 10 | 11 (55) | 10.7 (10-16) |
| III | 34 | 21 | 13 | 22 (64.7) | 6.8 (1-20) |
| IV | 66 | 38 | 28 | 37 (56) | 25.4 (2-35) |

Table 3. Pituitary adenomas classification according to their endocrine symptoms: Clinically functioning pituitary adenomas (F) and clinically non-functioning pituitary adenomas (NF). Prolactin hormone expression detected by immunohistochemistry (Prl). Number and percentage of positive cases, in each grade. Ki-67 Labeled Index (Ki-67-LI) in each grade. ND= No determined.

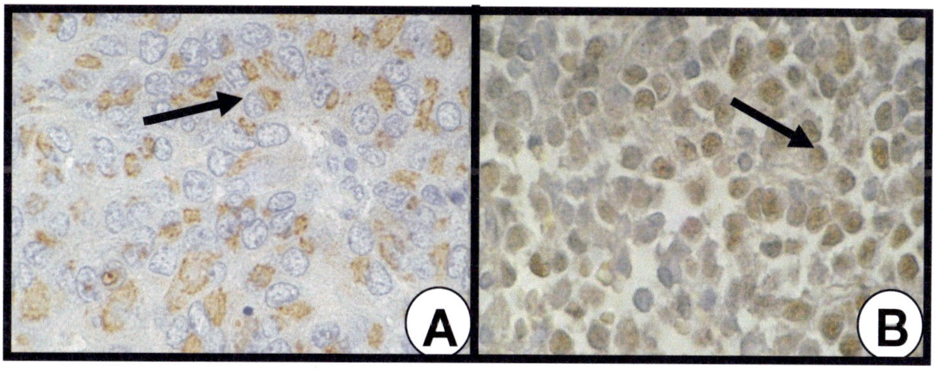


Fig. 3. Immunohistochemical detection

Photomicrograph of pituitary adenomas stained with immunohistochemical technique. Antibodies against prolactin hormone (A), and Ki-67 (B). Prolactin detection is present in the cytoplasm and Ki-67 can be seen in nucleus. Arrows show the immunodetection. (original magnification X 400).

### 3.2 Statistical analysis

There was no significative statistic difference in disease evolution time (F=1.0, p=0.351) and follow up (F=0.1, p=0.885), compared between invasion degrees. Neither the evolution time (p=0.146) nor the follow-up time (p=0.678) differed between functioning PA and non-functioning PA, however disease evolution time was lightly higher in III and IV invasion degrees. Evolution time ($X^2$=2.4, p=0.287) and follow up time ($X^2$=0.1, p=0.939) did not have association with the invasion grade.

No association was found among recurrence and functioning PA (p=0.526), and with hormone immunodetection (Prl p=0.595; GH p=0.377; FSH p=0.635).

Ki 67-LI was higher in IV grade (median value: 24.5%; range 2-35) in comparison with grade II (median value 6.8%; range 1-20; $X^2$=6.4, p=0.029); Grade III PA has an intermediate value (median value 10.7%; range 10-16). There was no statistic difference of Ki-67-LI between functioning PA and non-functioning PA (p=0.893) or between PA with recurrence and PA without recurrence (p=0.253). There was no association of Ki-67-LI with hormone secretion type (Prl p=0.121; GH p=0.100; FSH p=0.5).

### 3.3 Histopathological analysis

Histologically 98.4% show high cellular density, discrete nuclear pleomorphism, and dense nuclei, between 7 and 10 μ of diameter (Fig. 4A). Neither necrosis areas nor mitotic figures were observed. Only two cases of IV grade invasion degree, which were prolactin secretor PA, show nuclear pleomorphism, pseudoinclusions, bi- or multinucleated cells, and mitotic figures (Fig. 4B and 4C).

There were 11 prolactinomas (15.2%) treated with bromocriptine before surgery for a period of 2 months to 3 years. The drug decreased tumor size and serum prolactin levels, the menstruation was restored, galactorrhea stopped and fertility returned. Histologically interstitial fibroses was observed in these tumors (Fig. 4D). Ultrastructuraly the cells showed smaller endoplasmic reticulum and Golgi complex; lysosomes were more frequent observed and there were scarce secretory granules.

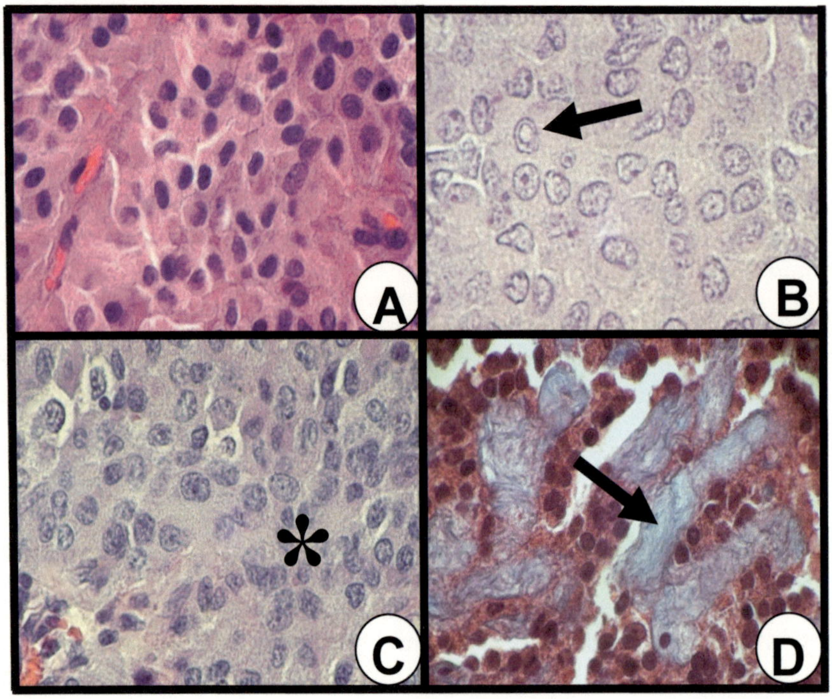


Fig. 4. Photomicrograph of pituitary adenomas with hematoxilyn-eosin stain (A-C), and with Masson's trichrome stain for collagen fibers (D). (A) PA showing solid pattern with homogeneous size cells. (B-C) PA showing nuclear pleomorphism (asterisk) and pseudoinclusions (arrow). (D) Bromocriptine treated PA which shows interstitial fibrosis (arrow). (Original magnification: X400).

### 3.4 Ultrastructure

#### 3.4.1 Prolactin adenomas

The most frequent type of pituitary adenomas was the prolactinoma (59%). All prolactinomas were sparsely granulated. The tumor show polyhedral cells with irregular nucleus, and prominent nucleolus. In the cytoplasm abundant, lamellar, rough endoplasmic reticulum and well development Golgi complex, was observed. There were scarce secretory granules, with size between 100-300 nm in diameter; some of them were localized between lateral cell surfaces which are known as misplaced exocytosis, the morphologic mark of prolactin secretor PA (Fig. 5).

#### 3.4.2 Growth hormone adenomas

Adenoma secreting only growth hormone had an incidence of 4%. Ultrastructuraly this tumor was sparsely granulated. The cells showed pleomorphic and eccentric nucleus, with scarce and dilated endoplasmic reticulum. Fibrous bodies with type II filaments were observed, some of them with secretory granules inside it, whose size was between 221 nm and up to 769 nm in diameter (Fig. 6A).

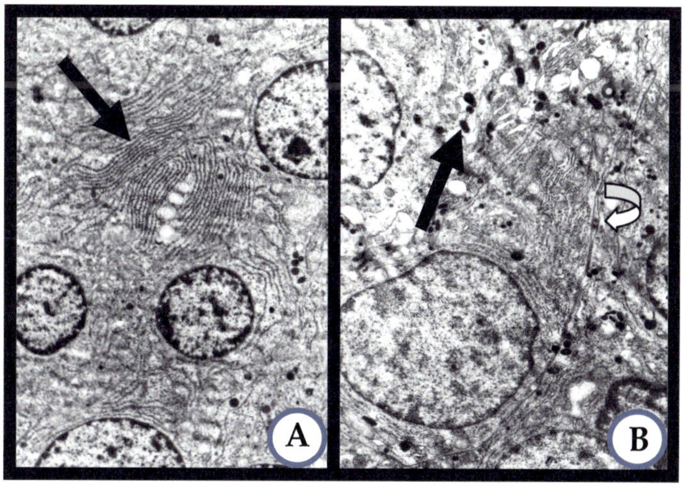


Fig. 5. Electronmicrographs of sparsely granulated prolactin adenoma grade II. (A) Lamellar endoplasmic reticulum (arrow). X 6,076; (B) fused secretory granules (black arrow) and misplaced exocytosis (white curved arrow). X9,750. Uranyl acetate-lead citrate.

### 3.4.3 GH secreting adenoma and prolactin hormone adenoma

Ten cases (8%) of pituitary adenomas with prolactin hormone and growth hormone secretion were found. Ultrastructuraly it was observed a monomorphous tumor, formed by only one cell type. All cells were scarcely granulated with secretory granules with 178 nm of diameter, few mitochondrias, lamellar endoplasmic reticulum and folded cell membranes;

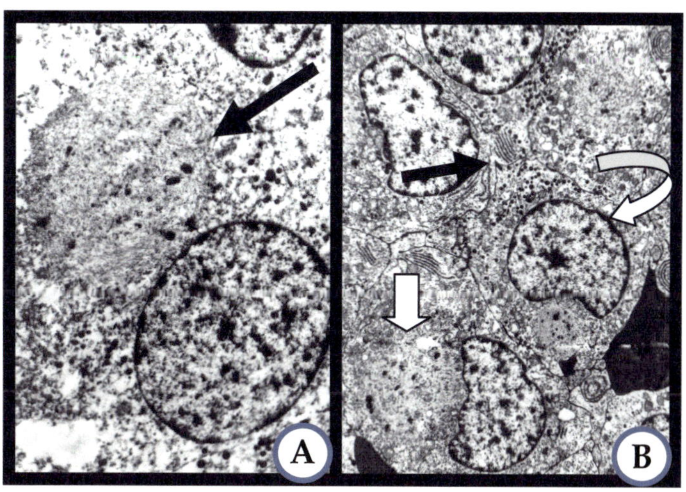


Fig. 6. Electronmicrograph of grade IV, GH PA, with their hall-mark fibrous body (arrow) X10,350. (A); grade III PA, prolactin and GH secreting, with lamellar endoplasmic reticulum (black arrow), crescent moon nuclei (curved arrow), and fibrous body of type II filaments (white arrow). X5,137. (B). Uranyl acetate-lead citrate.

nucleus show rounded or crescent moon shape in which concave area fibrous bodies were observed (Fig. 6B).

### 3.4.4 Gonadotroph adenomas

These adenomas were the most abundant (12%) after prolactinomas (44%) and the negative types for immunohistochemistry (21%). This tumor was formed by polyhedral cells, with poorly developed cytoplasm. Nuclei had rounded contours, some of them with irregular shapes and eccentric nucleoli attached to the electron-dense perinuclear chromatin. Rough endoplasmic reticulum was scarce and dilated, and secretory granules were few and small (153 nm in diameter). Big Golgi complex was observed with dilated cisterns (Fig. 7A). In two IV grade cases, smooth endoplasmic reticulum, mixed with mitochondria and pleomorphic secretory granules were detected; there was a vacuolated Golgi complex which was arranged in a honey comb complex, the hall-mark of this adenoma type (Fig. 7B).

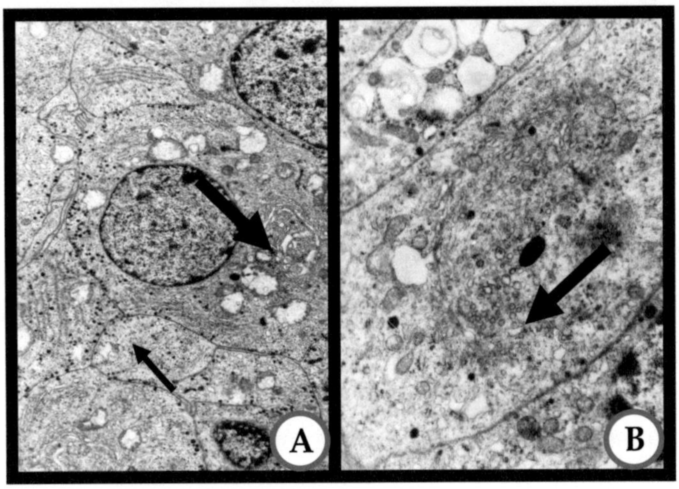


Fig. 7. Electronmicrograph of grade III gonadotroph PA. (A) This tumor showed big Golgi complex with dilated cisterns (arrow), small secretory granules located along the cell membrane (thin arrow). X 6,370; (B) Golgi shows a honey comb complex (arrow). X15,600. Uranyl acetate-lead citrate.

### 3.4.5 Negative pituitary adenomas

This type of tumors was negative for all hormones with the immunohistochemistry technique. Under transmission electron microscopy, poorly developed cells were observed with scarce rough endoplasmic reticulum, few secretory granules with 100-200 nm of diameter and small Golgi complex. In some cases it was observed numerous mitochondria, which is known as oncocytic transformation (Fig. 8A).

### 3.4.6 Corticotroph adenoma

There were 2 cases (1.6%) of ACTH secreting pituitary adenomas. This tumor showed polyhedral or elongated cells with poorly developed cytoplasm. The cell boundaries were clearly marked, elongated nuclei with irregular contours, and prominent nucleoli (8B);

secretory granules were scarce and small (104 nm). In one case proliferation of type I filaments were perceive with secretory granules inside it (Fig. 8C).

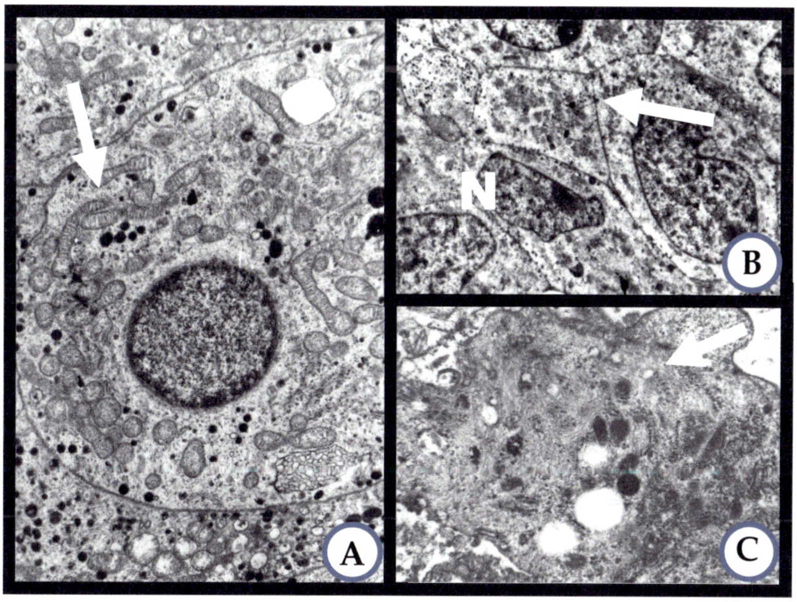


Fig. 8. (A) Electronmicrography of grade IV immunonegative PA. This tumor showed sparsely granulated cells with abundant mitochondria (arrow). X9,900 ; (B) Corticotroph cell adenoma grade III which consist of closely-apposed, angular cells, with marked cell boundaries (arrow), and nucleus with irregular shape (N). X6,370 ; (C) Cytoplasm with abundant type I filaments were observed (arrow). X8760. Uranyl acetate and lead citrate.

## 4. Discussion

Pituitary adenomas are heterogeneous tumors, this is because their different types of cells. The analysis of them had take into account several characteristic, the aim of these is to explain its behavior, although until now, has not been understood.

Pituitary adenomas comprise nearly 15% of intracranial neoplasms and are the most common lesions in the sellar region (Valassi et al., 2010). There is a report of 84.6% PA in a study of 4,122 tumors of sellar region (Saeger et al., 2007). In a 10-year study conducted at the National Institute of Neurology and Neurosurgery, in Mexico City, from 2,041 central nervous system tumors and covers, 26.2% were PA (personal communication). Here we present a study of 122 case of PA which occurred between 13 and 75 yr old, with peak of incidence from 20 and 60 years (100 cases; 81.9%), 10 yr earlier than other series (Davis et al., 2001). There was a slightly higher incidence in men; however women had earlier age at diagnosis (since 13 yr) than men (since 17), with higher frequency between 20 and 48 yr (men between 30 and 60 yr; 68%).

Pituitary adenomas incidence are rare in young people under 20 yr and mostly are prolactinomas (86%) or corticotropinomas (10%) (Mindermann & Wilson, 1994). In this study was found 12 patients under 20 yr (9.8%); Nine (75%) were prolactinomas, one of which was Prl-ACTH positive, two Prl-GH, one Prl-TSH. From these 12 cases, one (8.3%) was GH immunopositive and in 2 PA the hormone expression was no detected. In table 1 it can be observed, that in some patients the age at diagnosis (age column) is over 20 yr, although the patients reported that the beginning of the symptoms was some years before (evolution time).

In general, tumor size correlates with functional activity (clinically functioning and clinically non-functioning pituitary adenomas), and in women has been observed that, prolactinomas and also in ACTH clinically functioning pituitary adenomas, the diagnosis is carry out at early stages. (Kontogeorgos, 2006). In our work we found 71 (58.1%) functioning PA; 44 (61.9%) were in female of which only 5 (11%) were grade I and II PA and 39 (88.6%) were classified in III and IV grades. Out of this 39 PA, 29 (74%; 13 in grade III and 16 in grade IV) were prolactin immunopositive. In this case, women functioning adenomas, which produced prolactin hormone, were detected at an advance stage of invasion.

In this study must of the PA were in a invasive phase (grade III and IV), and the disease evolution time in these patients was higher than in I and II grades, even though there was no statistical association with clinical manifestation (functioning or non-functioning PA) or hormonal activity assessed by immunohistochemistry. Similar long evolution time (from 10 days to 20 years), has been reported in a Brazilian serie which was greater than the Italian and US series (Drange et al, 2000; Ferrante et al., 2006). This may be due to the class of population that assist to this Institute, which are used to endure the symptoms of the disease for a long time before seeking medical treatment, or do not have the right information to perceive them at an early stage, also before turning to adequate health service they look for alternative therapies. As it has been suggested by other authors, the clinical signs might be underestimated or not correctly diagnosed (Drange et al., 2000; Ferrate et al., 2006). In our experience, patients as first choice went to the ophthalmologist, because of the visual alterations, and by the computed tomography or magnetic resonance imaging scans, sellar alterations were observed. Nowadays incidental detection of PA tumors has been increased due to radiological evaluations performed for unrelated reasons (Saeger et al., 2007). In this analysis we can observed that the functionality was not related to tumor size, but with time the patient will assit to the health center.

Non-functioning pituitary adenomas are a diverse and heterogeneous group, where glycoprotein hormones, null cell adenoma and oncocytoma are included (Laws et al., 1982; Moreno et al., 2005). They are usually diagnosed as macroadenomas due to absence of clinical manifestations, which cause tumor growth in long time. Non-functioning PA account between 15% and 45% of pituitary tumors (Asa & Kovacs, 1992; Milker-Zabel et al., 2005). It has been reported that 95-100% of non-functioning pituitary adenomas are macroadenomas, and the frequency of recurrence varies between 19% and 34.8% in different studies (Aurer & Clarici, 1985; Reddy et al., 2011); up to 79% has hormone expression, evaluated by immunohistochemistry (Moreno et al., 2005), being gonadotroph hormones and/or their α- β- subunits the most common (Cury et al., 2009, Hanson et al., 2005). In our study 51 (42%) tumors were non-functioning PA, of which 38 (74.5%) were men, this is consistent with other studies (Asa & Kovacs, 1992; Cury et al., 2009; Ferrante et al., 2006; Milker-Zabel et al., 2005). Out of 51 non-functioning pituitary adenomas, 15 (29.4%) showed recurrence and 41 (80%) were macroadenomas. In 71% of non-functioning PA hormone expression was found, being prolactin the most frequent hormone detected by immunohistochemistry (33%), followed by gonadotroph hormones (20%); there were 29% of immunonegative PA in accordance with Turner report (Turner et al., 1999). It is important to point out that 13 cases of non-functionig PA were female, 7 of grade III and 6 of grade IV.

There were no adenomas classified in grades I and II. In our case, in women non-functioming pituitary adenomas could be related with the size.

In pituitary adenomas recurrences are common problems. The large size and the invasive behavior of these tumors cause difficulties in their removal (Paek et al., 2005). It has been reported that about 50% of patients have tumor remnants, and tumor re-growth can be presented at 10 years after neurosurgery (Reddy, 2011; Sassolas et al., 1993). Generally larger tumors recurred more frequently than smaller adenomas after surgery (Gopalan et al., 2011; Saeger et al., 2007). In our work the tumors were removed between 60% and 100%, by means of transcranial-frontal or transsphenoidal technique, and in III and IV grades the recurrences were higher, with secondary recurrences in 5 patients (three in III grade and 2 in IV grade). The time of interval between surgery and recurrence ranged from 1 to 11 years in both clinically functioning PA and non-functioning PA. In non-functioning pituitary adenomas Reddy et al. (2011) showed relapse/re-growth in 10 or more years after the initial surgery, and found significant increase in re-growth rates when remnant pituitary tumors are observed on the first post-operative scan or if the patient is younger age at initial surgery.

The follow up time of the patients is an important factor for their outcome (Dekkers et al., 2008). In our work 38 (31%) patients were found with a mean of 11 yr of follow up (range 1-27 yr), 12 of them were non-functioning PA with 10.3 yr of follow up (range, 1-27 yr). Reddy et.al. (Reddy, 2011) reports an average of 6.1 yr (range, 1-25.8) of follow up in 29 patients with non-functioning PA out of 155, of which 54 (34.8%) had recurrence, with 20% of relapse after 10 years of surgery; they suggest that it is necessary to track patients beyond this time.

In this study, few patients continued to attend for monitoring appointments. This could be because the patients who come to this health institution live outside of Mexico city, and sometimes it is difficult for them to travel to the city. Other patients are sent to other hospitals for continue their treatment, or they have no financial means for the follow up. Patients, who maintain their treatment and attendance to appointments for periodic reviews, have good outcome, with a improve of their visual impairments and hormonal levels, treated by hormonal substitution. It has been observed that patients with pre-operative anterior dysfunction recover function after surgery and the cases who presented with visual disturbance improve their vision with a second surgery (Chang et al., 2010; Müslüman et al., 2011).

An important factor in the biological behavior of pituitary adenomas is their proliferative capacity, which could be assessed by counting mitoses and the immunostaining of nuclei for proliferation markers as Ki-67. Mitoses figures are rare in non-invasive pituitary adenomas (3.9% of cases), they are more frequent in invasive PA (21.4%) and are greater in carcinomas (66.7%) (Pernicope et al., 2001). In our study there were found 2 cases (1.6%) with mitoses, which is not different from that reported in other studies, including the recently established rare subtype spindle cell oncocytoma of the pituitary gland (Matyja et al., 2010; Saeger et al., 2007).

Ki-67 is the most important proliferation marker; it is expressed in early G1, S, G2, and M phases of the cell cycle. This marker is associated with tumor proliferation, invasiveness, and prognosis (Cattoretti et al., 1992; Petrowsky et al., 2001). In pituitary adenomas the value of Ki-67 is controversial, in relation to the aggressive behavior (de Aguiar et al., 2010; Zhao et al., 1999), and in pituitary carcinoma appear to predict rapid disease progression (Dudziak et al., 2011). In a study performed in 44 pituitary macroadenomas, visual field defect and recurrence show correlation with Ki-67 LI, no statistical differences were observed in Ki-67 LI in relation to the Hardy´s classification (Paek et al., 2005). In other study in a series of 20 radically resected pituitary macroadenomas (11 functioning, 9 nonfunctioning) MIB-1(antibody of Ki-67 antigen) did not show a significant difference of expression between recurrent and non-recurrent adenomas (Ruggeri et al., 2011). Yarman (2010) assessed Ki-67 expression in growth hormone-secreting pituitary adenomas and showed no correlation with the invasive character. In other study it has been observed that Ki-67 LI was marginally higher in clinically functioning adenomas than clinically non-functioning adenomas. They also found significant difference in the MIB-1 LI in tumors with a maximum diameter of more than 4cm at a MIB-1 LI of ≥2%, however this difference was not statistically significant at a higher MIB-1 LI cut off value of >3% (Chacko et al., 2010). On the other hand, there is other report in which no significant difference in MIB-1 LI was found between functioning and non-functioning PA (Scheithauer et al., 2006). In our results, Ki-67 LI was significantly higher in IV grade PA than those of II grade which is different to that reported by Paek (2005); however there was no statistic difference of Ki-67 LI between pituitary adenomas with recurrence or without recurrence. About functionality we did not found differences between functioning and non-functioning pituitary adenomas which differs with Scheithauer report (2006).

Ultrastructural analysis of pituitary adenomas is an important tool for the detailed characterization of this type of tumors, particularly in problematic cases, because it is the initial basis of adenoma classification. With transmission electron microscopy it can be confirmed the endocrine nature of PA and their functional differentiation, which can be identified based on their ultrastructural markers of each hormonal type. Despite the utility of electron microscopy analysis in the evaluation of these tumors, diagnostic cannot be made on ultrastructural grounds alone, it should be done taking into consideration histology, immunohistochemistry and electron microscopical morphologic features, as well as findings from imaging studies and the symptoms (Kontogeorgos, 2006). Both clinical and histopathological factors are important for the diagnostic and outcome of patients.

In our study we observed the ultrastructural features of the different types of PA according to their hormonal expression, and in relation to clinical manifestations. Ultrastructural analysis was very useful in mixed secretory adenomas, as growth hormone and prolactin secreting PA where cells with fibrous bodies, hall-mark of GH pituitary adenoma. In this way, ultrastructural findings of most PA are consistent with the immunophenotype, however there are occasional cases with ultrastructural features less well differentiated like the rare carcinomas (Scheithauer et. al., 2001).

## 5. Conclusion

Pituitary adenomas are a heterogeneous group whose behavior has not been understood yet. In our study must of the tumors were in a extensive invasive phase, they affected young adult population and in this series of cases people under 20 years were founded. The disease evolution time and recurrence frequency was high in the advanced grades. The diagnosis of these tumors was not related with the clinical manifestations, according to the time taken by the patients to consult a doctor. The good outcome of patients depends on the follow-up, which has a very low rate for different reasons.

Pituitary adenomas have benign histological aspect, however can be aggressive, and may have one or more recurrences, as has been shown in this analysis. These neoplasms seem to have, a natural evolution, a potential to invasion, sparing the nervous tissue and without seeding to distant organs.

Although there are no parameters or experimental tests that serve as clear markers of disease progression, the data that have been obtained as a result of the evaluation of hormone expression and clinical evaluation, have important information that can be associated with pathogenicity of PA. Currently, there are new molecular techniques, as proteomic technique that allows us to investigate the proteins involved in the disease process.

The setup of registry on pituitary tumours constitutes a useful tool to analyze clinical experience, improve therapeutic strategies and patient's care. It also contributes for teaching medical students and develops clinical research.

## 6. References

Asa, S.L. & Kovacs, K. (1992). Clinically non-functioning human pituitary adenomas. *Can J Neurol Sci,* Vol.19, No.2 (May), pp.228–35, ISSN: 0317-1671.

Bratthauer G.L, Adams L.R. (1994). Immunohistochemistry: Antigen detection in tissue. In: Mikel UV (ed) Advanced laboratory methods in histology and pathology. Armed Forces Institute of Pathology, American Registry of Pathology, Washington DC.

Cattoretti, G.; Becker, M.H.; Key, G.; Duchrow, M.; Schlüter, C.; Galle, J. & Gerdes, J. (1992). Monoclonal antibodies against recombinant parts of the ki-67 antigen (MIB1 and MIB3) detect proliferating cells in micro-wave-processed formalin-fixed paraffin sections. *J Pathol,* Vol.168, No.4, (Dec), pp. 357-363, ISSN 1096-9896.

Chacko, G.; Chacko, A.G.; Kovacs, K.; Scheithauer, B.W.; Mani, S.; Muliyil, J.P. & Seshadri, M.S. (2010). The clinical significance of MIB-1 labeling index in pituitary adenomas. *Pituitary,* Vol.13, No.4, (Dec), pp. 337-344. ISSN 1573-7403.

Chang, E.F.; Sughrue, M.E.; Zada, G.; Wilson, C.B.; Blevins, L.S. Jr. & Kunwar, S. (2010). Long term outcome following repeat transsphenoidal surgery for recurrent endocrine-inactive pituitary adenomas. *Pituitary,* Vol.13, No.3, (Sep), pp. 223-229, ISSN 1573-7403.

Colao, A.; Ochoa, A.S.; Auriemma, R.S.; Faggiano, A.; Pivonello, R. & Lombardi G. (2010). Pituitary carcinomas. *Front Horm Res,* Vol.38, pp. 94-108, ISSN 1662-3762.

Couldwell, W.T. & Cannon-Albright, L. (2010). A heritable predisposition to pituitary tumors. *Pituitary,* Vol.13, No.2, (June), pp. 130–137, ISSN 1573-7403.

Crocker, D.W. (1978). The pituitary gland. En: Coulson W.F. (Ed): *Surgical Pathology,* pp. 878-898, Lippincott, Philadelphia, 1978.

Cury, M.L.; Fernandes, J.C.; Machado, H.R.; Elias, L.L.; Moreira, A.C. & Castro, M. (2009). Non-functioning pituitary adenomas: clinical feature, laboratorial and imaging assessment, therapeutic management and outcome. *Arq Bras Endocrinol Metabol,* Vol.5, No.1, (Feb), pp. 31-39, ISSN 1677-9487.

Davis, J.R.; Farrell, W.E. & Clayton, R.N. (2001). Pituitary tumours. *Reproduction* Vol.121, No.3, (Mar), pp. 363-371, ISSN 1741-7899.

de Aguiar, P.H.; Aires, R.; Laws, E.R.; Isolan, G.R.; Logullo, A.; Patil, C. & Katznelson L. (2010). Labeling index in pituitary adenomas evaluated by means of MIB-1: is there a prognostic role? A critical review. *Neurol Res,* Vol.32, No.10, (Dec), pp. 1060-1071, ISSN 1743-1328.

Dekkers, O.M.; Pereira, A.M. & Romijn, J.A. (2008). Treatment and follow-up of clinically nonfunctioning pituitary macroadenomas. *J Clin Endocrinol Metab*, Vol.93, No.10, (Oct), pp. 3717-3726, ISSN 1945-7197.

Drange, M.R.; Fram, N.R.; Herman-Bonert, V. & Melmed, S. (2000). Pituitary tumour registry: anovel clinical resourse. *J Clin Endocrinol Metab*, Vol.85, No.1, (Jan), pp. 168-174, ISSN 1945-7197.

Dudziak, K.; Honegger, J.; Bornemann, A.; Horger, M. & Müssig K. (2011). Pituitary carcinoma with malignant growth from first presentation and fulminant clinical course--case report and review of the literature. *J Clin Endocrinol Metab*, Vol. 96, No.9, (Sep), pp. 2665-2669, ISSN 1945-7197.

Ferrante, E.; Ferraroni, M.; Castrignanò, T.; Menicatti, L.; Anagni, M.; Reimondo, G.; Del Monte, P.; Bernasconi, D.; Loli, P.; Faustini-Fustini, M.; Borretta, G.; Terzolo, M.; Losa, M.; Morabito, A.; Spada, A.; Beck-Peccoz, P. & Lania, AG. (2006). Non-functioning pituitary adenoma database: a useful resourse to improve the clinical management of pituitary tumors. *Eur J Endocrinol*, Vol.155, No.6, (Dec), pp.823-829, ISSN 1479-683X.

Galland, F. & Chanson, P. 2009. Classification and pathophysiology of pituitary adenomas. *Bull Acad Natl Med*, Vol.193, No.7, (Oct), pp. 1543-1556, ISSN 0001-4079.

Gopala, R.; Schlesinger, D; Vance, M. L.; Laws, E. & Sheehan, J. (2011). Long-term outcomes after Gamma Knife radiosurgery for patients with a nonfunctioning pituitary adenoma. Neurosurgery, Vol.69, No.2, (Aug), pp. 284-93, ISSN 1524-4040.

Hanson, P.L.; Aylwin, S.J.B.; Monson, J.P,; Burrin, J.M. (2005). FSH secretion predominates in vivo and in vitro in patients with non-functioning pituitary adenomas. *European J of Endocrinol*, Vol.152, No.3, (Mar), pp.363–370, ISSN:1479-683X.

Hardy, J. (1973). Transsphenoidal surgery of hypersecreting pituitary tumors, In: Diagnosis and treatment of pituitary tumors. Int Congress Series No. 303. Edited by Kohler PO, Ross GT. Excerpta Medica; pp. 179-98. Amsterdam.

Horvath, E. & Kovacs K. (1992). Ultrastructural diagnosis of human pituitary adenomas. *Microsc Res Tech*, Vol.20, No.2, (Jan), pp. 107-35, ISSN 1097-0029.

Horvath, E. (1994). Ultrastructural markers in the pathologic diagnosis of pituitary adenomas. Ultrastruct Pathol, Vol.18, No.1-2, (Jan-Apr), pp. 171-179, ISSN 1521-0758.

Kaltsas, G.A.; Nomikos, P.; Kontogeorgos, G.; Buchfelder, M. & Grossman AB. (2005). Clinical review: diagnosis and management of pituitary carcinmomas. *J Clin Endocrinol Metab*, Vol.90, No.5, (May), pp. 3089-3099, ISSN 1945-7197.

Kovacs, K. & Horvath E. (1986). Pituitary adenomas. In Tumors of the pituitary gland. Edited by Washington: Armed Forces Institute of Pathology; 1986:57-93. Hartmann W.H, Sobin L.H. Second Series: Atlas of tumor Pathology, Fascicle 21.

Kontogeorgos, G. (2006). Predictive markers of pituitary adenoma behavior. *Neuroendocrinology* Vol.83, No.3-4, (Oct), pp.179–188, ISSN: 1423-0194.

Laws, E.R.; Ebersold, M.J. & Piepgras DG. (1982).The results of transsphenoidal surgery in specific clinical entities. In: Laws E.R, Randall R.V, Kern E.B, et.al. Manegement of pituitary adenomas and related lesions with emphasis on transsphenoidal microsurgery. New York, Appleton-Century-Crofts pp. 277-305.

Lau, Q.; Scheithauer, B.; Kovacs, K.; Horvath, E.; Syro, L.V. & Lloyd R. (2010). MGMT immunoexpression in aggressive pituitary adenoma and carcinoma. *Pituitary*, Vol.13, No.4, (Dec), pp. 367-79, ISSN 1573-7403.

Li-Ng, M. & Sharma M. (2008). Invasive pituitary adenoma. *J Clin Endocrinol Metab*, Vol.93, No.9, (Sept), pp. 3284-3285, ISSN 1945-7197.

Martínez A.J. (1986). The pathology of nonfunctional pituitary adenomas. *Semin Diag Pathol,* Vol.3, No.1, (Feb), pp.83-94, ISSN 0740-2570.

Matyja, E.; Maksymowicz , M.; Grajkowska, W.; Olszewski, W.; Zieliński, G. & Bonicki, W. (2010). Spindle cell oncocytoma of the adenohypophysis - a clinicopathological and ultrastructural study of two cases. *Folia Neuropathol,* Vol.48, No.3, pp.175-184, ISSN 1509-572X.

McDowell, B.D.; Wallace, R.B.; Carnahan, R.M.; Chrischilles, E.A.; Lynch, C.F. & Schlechte, J.A. (2011). Demographic differences in incidence for pituitary adenoma. *Pituitary,* Vol.14, No.1, (Mar), pp.23-30, ISSN 1573-7403.

Milker-Zabel, S.; Debus, J.; Thilmann, C.; Schlegel, W. & Wannenmacher M. (2001). Fractionated stereotactically guided radiotherapy and radiosurgery in the treatment of functional and nonfunctional adenomas of the pituitary gland. *Int J Radiat Oncol Biol Phys* Vol.50, No.5, (Aug), pp.1279-1286. ISSN: 1879-355X.

Mindermann, T. & Wilson C.B. (1994). Age-related and gender-related occurrence of pituitary adenomas. *Clinical Endocrinology,* Vol.41, No.3, (Sep), pp.359-364. ISSN: 0300-0664.

Moreno, C.S.; Evans, Chheng-Orn; Zhan, X.; Okor, M.; Desiderio, D.M. & Oyesiku, N M. (2005). Novel molecular signaling and classification of human clinically nonfunctional pituitary adenomas identified by gene expression profiling and proteomic analyses. *Cancer Res,* Vol.65, No.22, (Nov), pp.10214-10222, ISSN 1538-7445.

Müslüman, A.M.; Cansever, T.; Yılmaz, A.; Kanat, A.; Oba, E.; Çavuşoğlu, H.; Sirinoğlu, D. & Aydın Y. (2011). Surgical results of large and giant pituitary adenomas with special consideration of ophthalmologic outcomes. *World Neurosurg,* Vol.76, No.1-2, (Jul-Aug), pp. 141-148, ISSN 1878-8750.

Nosé, V.; Ezzat, S.; Horvath, E.; Kovacs, K.; Laws E., Lloyd, R.; Lopes, B. & Asa S. (2011) Protocol for examination of specimens from patients with primary pituitary tumors. *Arch Pathol Lab Med* Vol.135, No.5, (May), pp.640-646, 1543-2165.

Paek, K.I.; Kim, S.H.; Song, S.H.; Choi, S.W.; Koh, H.S.; Youm, J.Y. & Kim, Y. (2005). Clinical significance of Ki-67 laveling index in pituitary macroadenoma. J *Korean Med Sci,* Vol.20, No.3, (Jun), pp. 489-494, ISSN 1598-6357.

Pernicope, P.J. & Scheithauer, B.W. (2001). Invasive pituitary adenoma and pituitary carcinoma. In Diagnosis and management pituitary tumors. pp 369-386. Eds K Thapar, K.; K. Kovacs, B.W., Scheithauer and K.V Lloyd, Totowa N.J: Humana press 2001.

Petrowsky, H.; Sturm, I.; Graubitz, O.; Kooby, D.A.; Staib-Sebler, E.; Gog, C.; Köhne, C.H.; Hillebrand, T.; Daniel, P.T.; Fong, Y. & Lorenz, M. (2001). Relevance of Ki-67 antigen expression and K-ras mutation in colorectal liver metastases. *Eur J Surg Oncol,* Vol.27, No.1, (Feb), pp. 80-87, ISSN 1532-2157.

Prophet, E. & Arrignton J. (Eds.). (1992). Histotechnologyc methods. USA Armed Forces Institute of Pathology, ISBN 1-881041-00-X, Washington, D. C.

Reddy, R.; Cudlip, S.; Byrne, J.V.; Karavitaki, N. & Wass, J.A. (2011). Can we ever stop imaging in surgically treated and radiotherapy-naive patients with non-functioning pituitary adenoma? *Eur J Endocrinol,* Vol.165, No.5, (Nov), pp. 739-44, ISSN 1479-683X.

Rosai, J. (1989). Pituitary adenomas. In: *Ackerman´s Surgical Pathology.* Volume 2. 7th ed. Edited by Rosai J. St. Louis: C. V. Mosby;:1779-1789.

Ruggeri, R.M.; Costa, G.; Simone, A.; Campennì, A.; Sindoni, A.; Ieni, A.; Cavallari, V.; Trimarchi, F. & Curtò, L. (2011). Cell proliferation parameters and apoptosis indices in pituitary macroadenomas. *J Endocrinol Invest,* Sep 6. [Epub ahead of print] ISSN 1720-8386.

Saeger, W.; Lüdecke, D.K.; Buchfelder, M.; Fahlbusch, R.; Quabbe, H-J. & Petersenn, S. (2007). Pathohistological classification of pituitary tumors: 10 years of experience with the German pituitary tumor registry. *European J Endocrinol* Vol.156, No.2, (Feb), pp.203-216, ISSN 0804-4643.

Sassolas, G.; Trouillas,J.; Treluyer, C.; Perrin,G. (1993). Management of non-functioning pituitary adenomas. Acta Endocrinol (Copenh), Vol.129, pp. 21-26.

Scheithauer B.W, Kovacs K.T, Laws Jr E.R, Randall R.V. (1986) Pathobiology of invasive pituitary tumors with special reference to functional classification. *J Neurosurg* Vol.65, No.6, (Dec), pp. 733-744, ISSN 1933-0693.

Scheithauer, B.W.; Fereidooni, F.; Horvath, E.; Kovacs, K.; Robbins, P.; Tews, D.; Henry, K.; Pernicone, P.; Gaffrey, T.A. Jr.; Meyer, F.B..; Young, W.F. Jr.; Fahlbusch, R.; Buchfelder, M. & Lloyd, R.V. (2001). Pituitary carcinoma: an ultrastructural study of eleven cases. *Ultrastruct Pathol*, Vol.25., No.3, (May-Jun), pp. 227-242., ISSN 1521-0758.

Scheithauer, B.W. ; Kurtkaya-Yapicier, O. ; Kovacs, K.T. ; Young, Jr. W.F. & Lloyd R.V. (2005). Pituitary carcinoma: a clinicopathologycal review. Neurosurg, Vol.56, No.5, (May), pp. 1066-1074, ISSN 1524-4040.

Scheithauer, B.W.; Gaffey, T.A.; Lloyd, R.V.; Sebo, T.J.; Kovacs, K.T.; Horvath, E.; Yapicier, O.; Young, W.F. Jr.; Meyer, F.B.; Kuroki, T.; Riehle, D.L. & Laws, E.R Jr. (2006). Pathobiology of pituitary adenomas and carcinomas. *Neurosurgery*, Vol.59, No.2, (Aug), pp. 341-353, ISSN 1524-4040.

Tena-Suck, M.L.; Salinas-Lara, C.; Sánchez-García, A.; Rembao-Bojórquez, D. & Ortiz-Plata A. (2006). Late development of intraventricular papillary pituitary carcinoma after irradiation of prolactinoma. *Surgical Neurol*, Vol.66, No.5, (Nov), pp. 527-533, ISSN 1879-3339.

Tichomirowa, M.A.; Daly, A.F. & Beckers, A. (2009). Familial pituitary adenomas. *J Intern Med*, Vol.266, No.1, (Jul), pp. 5–18, ISSN 1365-2796.

Turner, H.E.; Stratton, I.M.; Byrne, J.V.; Adams, C.B. & Wass J.A. (1999). Audit of selected patients with nonfunctioning pituitary adenomas treated without irradiation- a follow-up study. *Clin Endocrinol*, Vol.51, No.3, (Sep), pp.281-284, ISSN 1365-2265.

Valassi, E.; Biller, B.M.; Klibanski, A. & Swearingen, B. (2010). Clinical features of non-pituitary sellar lesions in a large surgical series. *Clin Endocrinol (Oxf)*, Vol.73, No.6, (Dec), pp.798-807, ISSN 1423-0194.

Vandeva, S.; Jaffrain-Rea, M.L.; Daly, A.F.; Tichomirowa, M.; Zacharieva, S. & Beckers, A. (2010). The genetics of pituitary adenomas. *Best Pract Res Clin Endocrinol Metab*, Vol.24, No.3, (Jun), pp. 461-76, ISSN 1532-1908.

Yarman, S.; Kurtulmus, N.; Canbolat, A.; Bayindir, C.; Bilgic, B. & Ince, N. (2010). Expression of Ki-67, p53 and vascular endothelial growth factor (VEGF) concomitantly in growth hormone-secreting pituitary adenomas; which one has a role in tumor behavior ? *Neuro Endocrinol Lett*, Vol.31, No.6, pp. 823-828, ISSN 0172-780X.

Yu R, Melmed S. (2010).Pathogenesis of pituitary tumors. *Prog Brain Res*, Vol.182, pp. 207-27, ISSN 1875-7855.

Zada, G.; Woodmansee, W.W.; Ramkissoon, S.; Amadio, J.; Nose, V. & Laws E.R. (2011). Atypical pituitary adenomas: incidence, clinical characteristics, and implications. *J Neurosurg*, Vol. 114, No.2, (Feb), pp. 336-44, ISSN 1933-0693.

Zhao, D.; Tomono, Y. & Nose, T. (1999). Expression of P27, Kip 1 and Ki-67 in pituitary adenomas: An investigation of marker of adenoma invasiveness. *Acta Neurochir (Wien)*, Vol.141, No.2, pp. 187-192, ISSN 0942-0940.

5

# Stereotactic Radiosurgery for Pituitary Adenomas

Ricardo H. Brau and David Lozada
*University of Puerto Rico / Medical Sciences Campus/ Department of Surgery/ Neurosurgery Section*
*Puerto Rico*

## 1. Introduction

Stereotactic Radiosurgery (SRS) is a technology that utilizes externally generated ionizing radiation to treat (a) defined target(s) in the head or spine without the need to make an incision. The target is defined by high-resolution stereotactic imaging. It uses multiple convergent beams aimed to the target. The beams deliver a maximal dose to the target (with precision of less than 1mm), while minimizing irradiation of the surrounding tissues. The treatment is performed in a single session. The procedure requires a multidisciplinary team consisting of a neurosurgeon, radiation oncologist and medical physicist. Technologies that are used to perform SRS include linear accelerators, particle beam accelerators and multisource Cobalt 60 units. In order to enhance precision, various devices may incorporate robotics and real time digital imaging. (*Stereotactic Radiosurgery Task Force AANS/CNS/ASTRO, March 20, 2006*).

"Stereotactic Radiosurgery" was invented by the Swedish neurosurgeon Lars Leksell in 1951. Since its introduction, stereotactic radiosurgery (SRS) has evolved from an investigational concept into a recognized neurosurgical procedure for the management of a wide variety of brain disorders. Currently, radiosurgery can be employed as an adjuvant or definite treatment modality for pituitary adenomas.

The three major sources of radiation used today to perform SRS are the multi-source Cobalt 60 units, modified linear accelerators and the particle beam accelerators. These machines provide extremely accurate targeting and precise treatment for brain tumors. They treat brain tumors and other cerebral conditions in a one-day treatment. The original system is the Gamma Knife® System (GKS). Its clinical efficacy has been well documented, with more than 550,312 cases treated worldwide by December 2009 providing the data for over 2,500 publications in peer-reviewed medical literature. The GKS is ideal for tumors less than 3.5 cm, and functional disorders of the brain.

The modified linear accelerator (m-LINAC) based radiosurgery machines are prevalent throughout the world. The modified linear accelerator systems use similar principles as the GKS to treat the patient, but the source of the radiation is a linear accelerator. Modified Linear accelerator-based radiosurgery generally utilizes a stereotactic head-frame, floor-stand and a 6-megavolt (MV) linear accelerator. The linear accelerator systems utilize radiation beams that are redirected in many "arcs" centered over an isocenter to lessen the adverse effects on healthy tissue. These machines can perform radiosurgery on tumors smaller than 3.5cm in diameter with the same range of precision of the GKS. Most of the GKS and m-LINAC systems employ a stereotactic head frame (ring). The head frame allows a precise localization of the lesion to be treated. The head frame, which is attached to the skull with four small screws, ensures that the radiation beams are precisely targeted. The frame also prevents head motion during the treatment procedure, which ensures that only the target area receives the prescribed radiation. However, modern localization techniques using bony landmarks identified by diagnostic X-Rays system has allowed some systems of m-LINAC to avoid the use of the stereotactic head frame. One of the advantages of these systems is that patients can be treated over more than one day without the need of wearing a head frame over extended periods of time, and in a few special situations can treat tumors slightly larger than 3.5 cm in diameter with this hypofractionating technique. Another advantage of the m-LINAC system is that they can use Intensity-Modulated Radiation Therapy (IMRT) and Image Guided Radiotherapy (IGRT) dosimetries algorithms to treat critically located lesions. In IMRT, the intensity of the radiation beam is non-uniform (i.e., modulated) across the treatment field, rather than producing a single, uniform, intensity beam. When combining this technique with the imaging done in the pre-plan, it further improves the delivery of radiation. These systems can provide treatment to lesions outside the brain.

A special type of m-LINAC is the CyberKnife® Robotic Radiosurgery System. It utilizes a 6 MV compact linear accelerator mounted on a computer-controlled six-axis robotic manipulator that permits a wide range of beam orientations and takes advantage of intelligent robotics to enable the effective treatment of tumors in the brain and anywhere in the body. To date, an estimated over 80,000 patients have been treated with the CyberKnife® System and currently more than 50 percent of all CyberKnife® procedures in the United States are extra cranial.

The proton beam radiosurgery systems employ a stream of protons to treat lesions. As of June 2011, there were a total of 37 proton therapy centers in Canada, China, England, France, Germany, Italy, Japan, Korea, Poland, Russia, South Africa, Sweden, Switzerland, and USA and more than 73,800 patients had been treated (Particle Therapy Co-Operative Group, 2011). One hindrance to universal use of the proton in cancer treatment is the size and cost of the cyclotron or synchrotron equipment necessary to produce the protons.

The authors have used a modified linear accelerator-based system to provide radiosurgery treatment to pituitary adenomas. The initial radiosurgery system installed in 1999 was manufactured by Radionics®. In 2003 this system was upgraded to a Brain Lab System® that incorporated a multileaf collimator.

## 2. The radiobiology of radiosurgery

The basic principle of ionizing radiation is the creation of ions or free radicals in the irradiated tissues. This ions or free radicals interact with the cell's molecules producing damage to them. The radiation dose is usually measured in grays, where one gray (Gy) is the absorption of one joule per kilogram of mass. These ions and radicals, which may be formed from the water and oxygen in the cell or from the tissue substance, can produce irreparable damage to DNA, proteins, membranes, and lipids that can evolve into the cell's death. The radiation effects can be seen in the order of minutes to years (Figure 1).

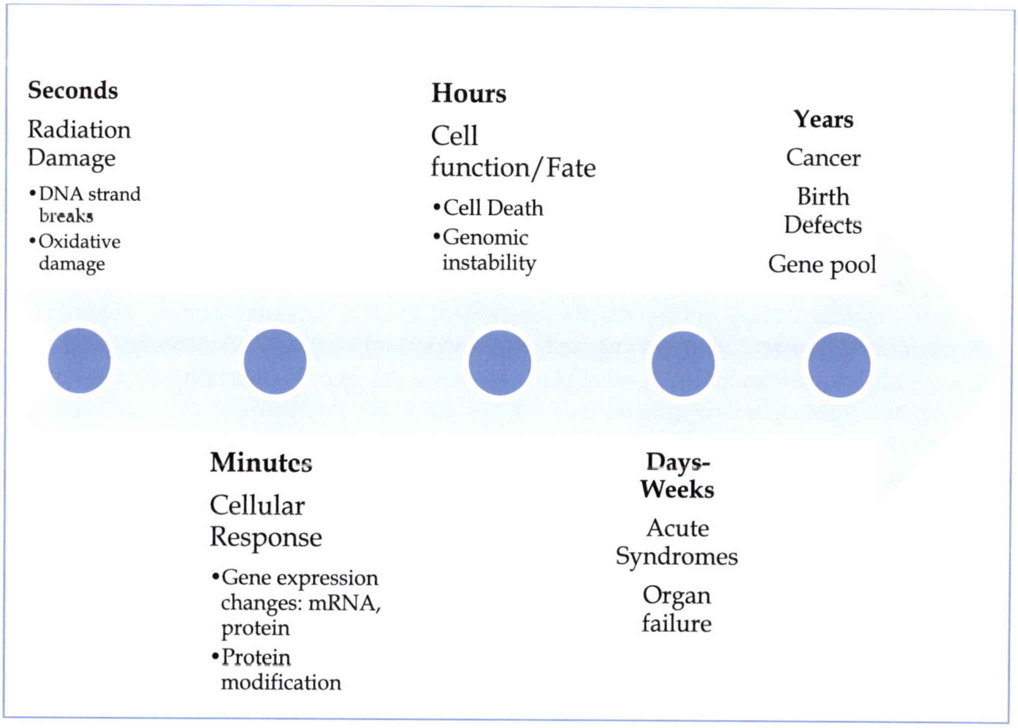


Fig. 1. Effects of Ionizing radiation over time.

Radiation damages the cell's structures of tumor cells as well of normal cells in the radiation beam path. Normal tissue, however, is generally more proficient repairing sublethal damage than tumors cells. In general terms, tumors cells have altered repair mechanisms tolerating less irradiation damage than normal cells. Cells require time to repair DNA damage and one of the normal responses of the cell is delaying the cell cycle, delaying G2 phase. In radiotherapy where daily treatments with sublethal doses of radiation are given for several days, the difference in proficiency to repair the damage between normal and tumoral tissues is essential. Therefore, the radiobiology of the cell cycle and differences in cell repair are of great importance for fractionated radiotherapy. In radiosurgery, were a lethal dose of radiation is given in a single treatment, the repairing capacity of different tissues play a less critical role. Radiosurgery in many instances activates the apoptosis cascade resulting in cell death. The rate of proliferation of cells can determine the response to radiation, resulting in increased sensitivity of endothelial, glial and subependymal cells. Vascular endothelial cell damage tends to produce vessels obliteration that could play a role in the death of tumor cells as well.

The radiation doses prescribed for radiotherapy have been developed from decades of clinical experience. However, the radiobiological principles of multifraction treatments do not necessarily apply to high dose ionizing beams as used in radiosurgery. Radiosurgery specifies a precise delivery of a high single fraction dose of ionizing beams to a defined target volume. Normal tissue is excluded from the target as much as possible and a steep dose gradient at the margin of the target volume assures that the surrounding tissue receives a minimal dosage. Therefore, repair capacity of normal tissue during treatment is less critical in radiosurgery.

## 3. Pituitary adenomas

Pituitary adenomas represent nearly 10-20% of all intracranial tumors. Multimodal treatment includes microsurgery, medical management, radiotherapy and radiosurgery. Pituitary adenomas are broadly classified into two groups—functioning (secretory) and nonfunctioning. Microsurgery is the primary recommendation for nonfunctioning and most of functioning adenomas, except for prolactinomas that are usually managed with dopamine agonist drugs. Long-term tumor control rates after microsurgery alone range from 50 to 80%. For both functioning and nonfunctioning pituitary adenomas, incomplete tumor resection or recurrence because of tumor invasion into surrounding structures (for example, the dura mater or cavernous sinus) is common. Postsurgical residual secretory adenoma results in the persistence of a hypersecretory state and the associated deleterious clinical features. Moreover, about 30% of patients require additional treatment after microsurgery for recurrent or residual tumors. In patients with recurrent or residual pituitary adenomas, treatment options include repeat resection, radiation therapy, medical management, and radiosurgery. More recently, radiosurgery has been established as a treatment option. Radiosurgery allows the delivery of prescribed dose with high precision strictly to the target and spares the surrounding tissues. Therefore, the risks of hypopituitarism, visual damage and vasculopathy are significantly lower. Furthermore, the latency of the radiation response after radiosurgery is substantially shorter than that of fractionated radiotherapy.

## 4. Planning and technique

All patients suspected of harboring a pituitary tumor should undergo a complete neurologic, ophthalmologic, endocrinologic, and radiologic work-up (Laws & Sheehan, 2006; Laws & Thapar 1996). This includes formal visual fields, an acuity testing and a detailed fundoscopic examination. Each facet of the hypothalamic-pituitary-end organ axis should be assessed by an endocrinologist and re-assessed by the neurosurgeon. (Table 1)

Evaluation of the sellar region is best accomplished by using a thin slice pre- and post-contrast magnetic resonance (MR) imaging. When there is a contraindication to MR or is not available, a computed tomography (CT) imaging can be useful (Jagannathan et al., 2005; Kanter et al., 2005).

If a patient has a neurological deficit attributable to an adenoma, surgery is the initial treatment of choice for all tumors except prolactinomas. Transsphenoidal microsurgery (endoscopic or microscopic) affords the best chance of rapid relief of mass effect and reduction in excessive hormone levels in patients with Cushing's disease and acromegaly (Laws & Sheehan, 2006; Laws & Thapar 1996; Laws et al., 1985a, 1985b, 2000). This approach is associated with a low rate of complications in the hands of experienced neurosurgeons (Ciric, 1997). For this reason, tumors located in areas such as the sellar floor or sphenoid that can be safely accessed surgically should undergo surgical removal, with radiosurgery being reserved for tumor residuals or recurrences. For tumors that cannot be removed completely depending on the size, location, and invasiveness of surrounding tissues by the tumor, one surgical goal could be to create a safe distance of 2 to 5 mm between the lesion and optic apparatus so that an adequate radiosurgery dose can be delivered to the adenoma with minimal risk of radiation injury to the optic pathways.

| Hormone | Test | Results and Additional Evaluations |
|---|---|---|
| Prolactin function | Serum Levels | Elevated prolactin, usually with serum levels > 75 ng/ml |
| Thyroid function | Free thyroxine and thyroid stimulating hormone | |
| Adrenal function | Morning fasting and afternoon serum cortisol and ACTH level. Salivary cortisol levels. | In Cushing's syndrome, a 24 h urine free cortisol and a dexamethasone suppression test. |
| Growth Hormone (GH) | Growth hormone and insulin-like growth factor (IGF)-1. | Oral glucose tolerance test with growth hormone measurements for GH secreting tumors. |

Table 1. Minimal basic endocrine workup for pituitary adenomas.

Patients harboring secretory pituitary tumors warrant a special consideration regarding radiosurgery pre-planning. Since 2000, several studies have documented that cessation of suppressive medication before radiosurgery is recommended to offer the best normalization of hormone values after the treatment (Landolt 2000a, 2000b, Pouratian et al., 2006, Pollock et al., 2007). The optimal time period to temporarily halt anti-secretory medications is unclear and class I evidence is sill unavailable to support temporary cessation of antisecretory medications as a standard of care.

## 5. Radiosurgery procedure

When medical and surgical treatments are not curative or cannot control the tumor growth or symptoms, radiosurgery needs to be considered. Prior to considering radiosurgery, the neurosurgeon and the radiation oncologist of the radiosurgery team evaluate the patient, both need to agree that radiosurgery is an optimal option. Then, the patient is scheduled for the procedure. On the day of the treatment or the day before, a MR study is obtained, with 3 mm thick slices of the brain including the sella and skull base. On the day of treatment a stereotactic head frame is applied under local anesthesia and/or IV sedation. Subsequently, stereotactic CT scanning is performed with the CT scan localizer on. Three-millimeter thick slices are obtained throughout the entire head. The stereotactic CT scan and MR images are transferred to the treatment-planning computer. The CT scan and MR images are fused electronically. The tumor, optic apparatus and critical surrounding structures are delineated in the planning computer. (Figure 2) The plan is carefully examined and adjusted to generate the actual treatment plan, maximizing the dose delivery to the tumor and minimizing irradiation of the optic apparatus and the surrounding tissues.

The radiation oncologist and the neurosurgeon review and approve the plan. Four or more sagittally oriented irradiation arcs are typically delivered using multileaf collimators. The multileaf collimator is adjusted every 15 degrees to achieve a conformal treatment to the lesion. The head ring is removed on the same day of treatment. After a short observation period, the patient is discharged. Close clinical and radiological neuroimaging follow-up examination is arranged at appropriate intervals depending on the entity treated and the condition of the patient.

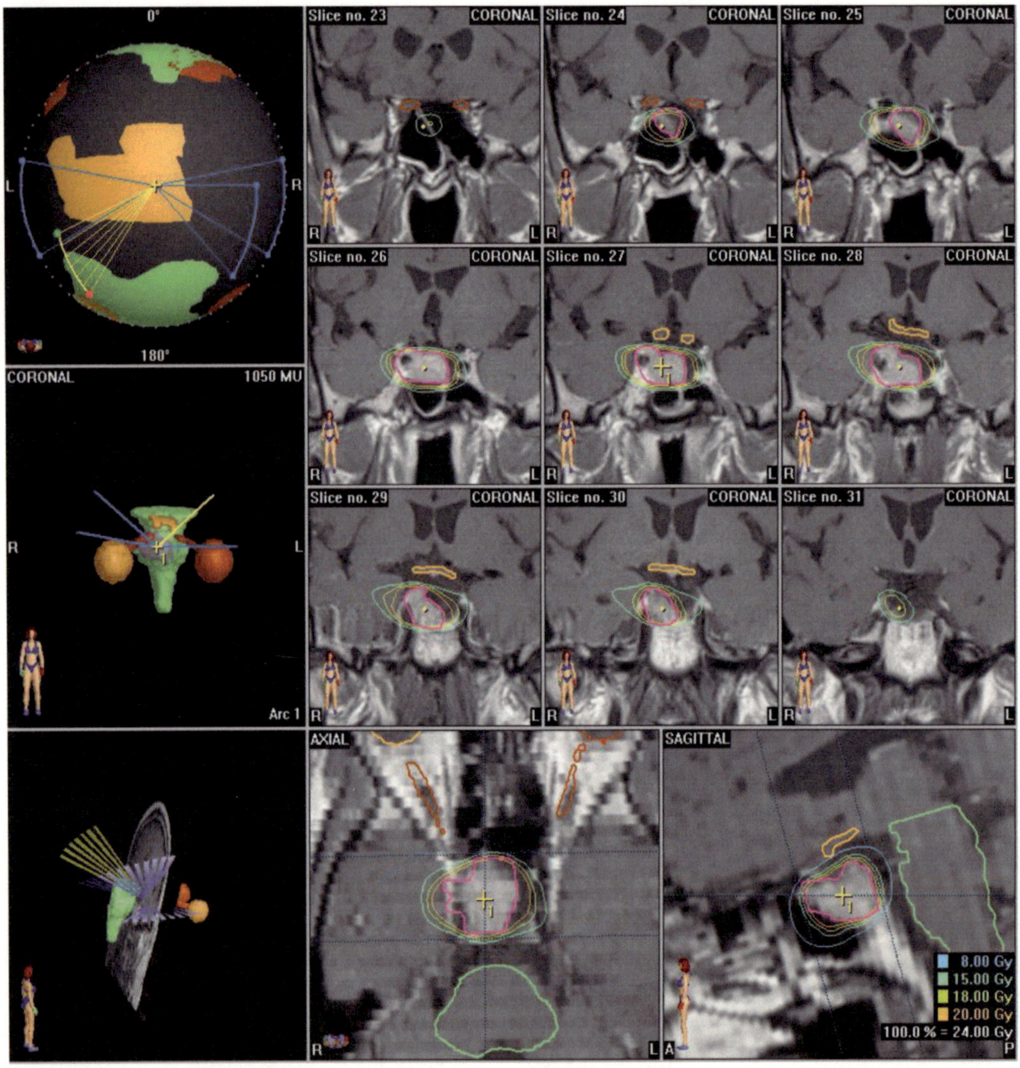


Fig. 2. Radiosurgical planning which includes protection of important structures and inclusion of treatment area.

## 6. Toxicity and side effects

Like any other medical intervention radiosurgery has side effects. The main concern is radionecrosis of structures adjacent to the pituitary gland; optic apparatus, cranial nerves within the cavernous sinus, hypothalamus, brainstem and medial temporal lobes. The toxicity of fractionated external beam radiotherapy is low; with 1.5% risk of radiation optic neuropathy (Brada et al., 1993; Tsang et al., 1994) and 0.2% risk of necrosis of normal brain structures (Becker et al., 2002). The most frequent late consequence of radiation is hypopituitarism likely to be primarily due to hypothalamic injury or primary pituitary gland injury. In patients with normal pituitary function around the time of radiotherapy, hormone replacement therapy is required in 20–40% of patients at 10 years. A rare late effect of radiation for pituitary adenoma is the development of second radiation-induced brain tumor. The reported frequency is in the region of 2% at 10–20 years (Brada et al., 1992; Tsang et al., 1993; Erfurth et al., 2001). Although there is an increased incidence of cerebrovascular accidents and excess cerebrovascular mortality in patients with pituitary adenoma treated with radiation, the influence of radiation on its frequency is not well defined (Brada et al., 1999, 2002; Tomlinson et al., 2001; Erfurth et al., 2002).

The radiation effects on the optic apparatus, other cranial nerves and brainstem are of critical importance. Most of the damage is thought to be a result of secondary damage of the endothelium of small vessels and protective Schwann cells or oligodendroglia. There is a difference in the tolerance of different cranial nerves; with sensory nerves (optic and acoustic) tolerating the least radiation. The nerves in the parasellar region, the facial nerves and the lower cranial nerves usually tolerate higher doses. Clinical experience suggests that these specialized sensory nerves do not show a great capacity to recover from injury. Although the precise dose tolerance of the cranial nerves is unclear, the anterior visual pathways seem to be the least radio-resistant, and single doses above 8 Gy should be avoided (Jagannathan et al., 2007; Leber et al., 1995, 1998). To minimize the risk of irradiation injuries to the optic apparatus, the distance between optic nerves and chiasm and the lesion being treated should be carefully assessed. A distance of 5 mm between the tumor and the optic apparatus is ideal, but a distance of as little as 2 mm may be acceptable. It appears that the risk may be related to the volume of the optic apparatus receiving the dose (Chen et al., 2001; Lim et al., 1998; Sheehan et al., 2000; Witt et al., 1998). However, a specific critical volume has not been agreed. This distance is critical to design a dose plan that delivers a lethal radiation dose to the tumor yet spare the optic apparatus. When all these precautions and considerations are taken care the patient is treated accordingly.

## 7. Radiosurgery for pituitary adenomas

The goals of radiosurgery for pituitary tumors are control of tumor growth, and in secretory adenomas to normalize hormonal hypersecretion. In addition to the above mention, these goals need to be carried out avoiding acute and delay radiation injury to neural structures and preventing secondary tumor formation.

### 7.1 Non-secreting tumors

In our experience of twelve patients treated for nonfunctioning pituitary tumors (with mean follow-up of 47 months), tumor volume decreased in three patients (25%), remained unchanged in eight (66%), and there was no increased in size. One patient was lost to follow-up. Regarding tumor control, eleven patients achieved tumor control (91%) except for the patient who was lost to follow-up. All of our patients were treated with LINAC Radiosurgery as secondary therapy. The average prescription peripheral dose (Gy) was 15.8Gy with a range from 8 to 22.5Gy. This is similar to previously published data. The median time of tumor shrinkage on MR-imaging was 12 months (range, 8-68 months) following radiosurgery. This is consistent with a recently published series that demonstrated pituitary adenomas were 90%, 80%, and 70% of their initial volume at 1, 2, and 3 years post-GK radiosurgery (Sheehan et al., 2002). Tumors involving the parasellar space require special consideration, as they would be otherwise untreatable.

Most other contemporary series involving stereotactic radiosurgery for non-functioning tumors (Table 2) have demonstrated excellent control of tumor growth, with a mean tumor control rate of 95.6% (range, 87%–100%) (Hayashi et al., 1999; Losa et al., 2004; Mitsumori et al., 1998; Morky et al., 1999; Muramatsu et al., 2003; Pollock & Carpenter, 2003; Pollock et al., 2008; Sheehan et al., 2002; Witt et al., 1998;).

In patients with four or more years of follow-up, the reported mean control rate is 95% (range, 83–100%) (Yoon et al., 1998; Morky et al., 1999; Feigl et al., 2002; Hoybye et al., 2001; Ikeda et al., 2001; Kobayashi et al., 2002; Shin et al., 2000; Wowra et al., 2002). Some series have even demonstrated improvement in visual function following radiosurgery after shrinkage of the tumor (Abe et al., 2002; Chen et al., 2001; Hayashi et al., 2005; Yoon et al., 1998). Nevertheless, prevention of tumor growth, without volume reduction, is still considered a radiosurgical goal.

The CyberKnife (Accuray, Calif., USA), is a newer radiosurgical device that is mounted on a maneuverable robotic manipulator and tracks the target with the aid of real-time guidance (Adler et al., 1997; Chang et al., 1998). Early experience with the Cyberknife has been promising for nonfunctioning adenomas, with a growth control rate of 95%, and lower prescription doses (14–16 Gy) than described for the Gamma Knife, although long-term clinical follow-up is still lacking (Kajiwara et al., 2005).

| Authors and Year | Radiosurgery Unit | No. of Patients | Mean/Median FU (months) | Max Dose (Gy) | Tumor Margin Dose(Gy) | Growth Control (%) |
|---|---|---|---|---|---|---|
| Mitsumori, et al., 1998 | LINAC | 7 | 47 | 19 | 15 | 100 |
| Witt, et al., 1998 | GK | 24 | 32 | 38 | 19 | 94 |
| Yoon, et al., 1998 | LINAC | 8 | 49 | 21 | 17 | 96 |
| Hayashi, et al., 1999 | GK | 18 | 16 | NR | 20 | 92 |
| Mokry, et al., 1999 | GK | 31 | 21 | 28 | 14 | 98 |
| Sheehan, et al., 2002 | GK | 42 | 31 | 32 | 16 | 98 |
| Muramatsu, et al., 2003 | LINAC | 8 | 30 | 26.9 | 15 | 100 |
| Pollock & Carpenter, 2003 | GK | 33 | 43 | 36 | 16 | 97 |
| Losa, et al., 2004 | GK | 54 | 41 | 33 | 17 | 96 |
| Iwai 2004 | GK | 34 | 60 | | 14 | 87 |
| Mingione 2006 | GK | 90 | 45 | | 18.5 | 92 |
| Pollock 2008 | GK | 62 | 45 | | 16 | 97 |
| Brau 2011* | LINAC | 12 | 47 | 21.7 | 15.8 | 91 |

Table 2. Summary of cases treated with Radiosurgery on Non-functioning pituitary adenomas. (*Unpublished manuscript in writing)

### 7.2 Secretory tumors

Most published results on radiosurgery for secretory adenomas have differed based on methodology, endocrine criteria for remission, the study population and length of follow-up. Most series typically report a higher prescription (margin) dose to patients with functioning adenomas, with a range between 20 Gy and 25 Gy in most reports (Jagannathan et al., 2007; Kim et al., 1999a, 1999b; Pouratian et al., 2006). Because hormone normalization has been followed in some cases by relapse, we prefer the term "remission" to "cure."

#### 7.2.1 Acromegaly

In our experience of fifteen patients treated for acromegaly (with mean follow-up of 37.2 months), tumor volume decreased in five patients (33.3%), remained unchanged in nine (60%), and there was one (6.6%) patient that showed an increase in tumor size. Tumor control was achieved in fourteen (93.3%) patients. All of our patients were treated with LINAC Radiosurgery as secondary therapy. The average prescription peripheral dose (Gy) was 19.4Gy with a range from 12 to 25Gy. In our experience, the rate of hormone normalization after radiosurgery for Acromegaly was seen in six (41.6%) patients. Hormone normalization in these five patients was observed at mean follow-up of 28 months. Tumor control was achieved in most patients correlating with hormone remission, except for one patient, which despite hormone remission there was a slight increase in tumor size.

The most widely accepted guidelines for endocrine remission in acromegaly consist of a GH level less than 1 ng/ml in response to an oral glucose challenge and a normal serum IGF-1 when matched for age [Giustina et al., 2000; Vance, 1998)

Published remission rates following radiosurgery for acromegaly vary widely from 0% to 100%, with the majority of patients achieving tumor growth control (Table 3) (Buchfelder et al., 1991; Cozzi et al., 2001; Freda, 2003; Fukuoka et al., 2001; Horvath et al., 1983; Landolt et al., 1998, 2000; Pouratian et al., 2006; Witt et al., 1998). Jezkova et al. reported a remission rate of 50% at 42 months follow-up in 96 patients with acromegaly who received

| Author and Year | RSx Unit | Pt No | F/U (mos) | Peripheral Dose (Gy) | IGF-1 Normalization (%) | Tumor Control (%) |
|---|---|---|---|---|---|---|
| Muramatsu, 2003 | LINAC | 4 | 30 | 15 | 50 | 100 |
| Attanasio 2003 | GK | 30 | 46 | 20 | 23 | 100 |
| Castinetti 2005 | GK | 82 | 49.5 | 12-40 | 40 | NR |
| Voges 2006 | LINAC | 64 | 54.3 | 15.3 | 49.8 | 97 |
| Jezkova 2007 | GK | 96 | 53.7 | 32 | 50 | 100 |
| Pollock 2007 | GK | 46 | 63 | 20 | 50 | 100 |
| Vik-Mo 2007 | GK | 53 | 66 | 26.5 | 58 | 89 |
| Losa 2008 | GK | 83 | 69 | 21.5 | 60.2 | 98 |
| Jagannathan 2008 | GK | 95 | 57 | 22 | 53 | 98 |
| Brau 2011* | LINAC | 15 | 37.2 | 19.4 | 41.6 | 93.3 |

Table 3. Summary of cases treated with Radiosurgery for Acromegaly. (*Unpublished manuscript in writing)

radiosurgery (Jezkova et al., 2006). Nearly one-third of these patients, however, had radiosurgery as primary treatment, without surgical extirpation of the adenoma. Pollock et al., (2007) demonstrated a remission rate of 50% in 46 patients with a higher remission rate in patients who were off suppressive medications at the time of radiosurgery. Pollock's group also stated that maximal radiosurgery effects may be delayed up to 5 years after treatment, therefore no other surgical treatment or additional radiosurgery should be considered within that period unless there is unequivocal evidence of tumor enlargement and progressive elevation of HGH and ILGF-1.

### 7.2.2 Cushing's disease

Cushing's disease is one of the most devastating pituitary disorders, and is associated with significant morbidity and premature death. Even after transsphenoidal surgery, up to 30% of patients may have persistent o recurrent disease (Ciric et al., 1997; Laws & Thapar, 1996; Mampalam et al., 1988). Most centers define an endocrine remission as a urine free-cortisol (UFC) level in the normal range associated with the resolution of clinical stigmata or a series of normal post-operative serum cortisol levels obtained throughout the day (Nieman, 2002; Sheehan et al., 2000). We have treated ten patients with Cushing's disease, with 40% of patients achieving normalization of hormones levels with a mean margin dose of 20.7Gy. The rate of remission statistically correlated with tumor volume, but not with tumor invasion into the cavernous sinus or the suprasellar region.

In our experience, the rate of hormone normalization after radiosurgery for Cushing's disease is difficult to predict, with remission occurring as early as 17months and as late as five years after LINAC Radiosurgery. Most patients who have remission, however, will do so within the first 2-3 years following radiosurgery. Patients with persistent disease should thus consider alternative treatments such as repeat TSS, or repeat radiosurgery (although this may be associated with a higher rate of cranial nerve damage) (Jagannathan et al., 2007).

Published endocrine remission rates following radiosurgery (Table 4) vary considerably, from 10% to 100%, with higher remission rates when radiosurgery follows surgical debulking (Arnaldi et al., 2003; Chu et al., 2001; Izawa et al., 2000; Jackson & Noren, 1999;

| Author and Year | RSx Unit | Pt No | F/U (mos) | Peripheral Dose (Gy) | Hormone Normalization (%) | Tumor Control (%) |
|---|---|---|---|---|---|---|
| Laws 1999 | LINAC | 50 | --- | 22 | 58 | --- |
| Izawa 2000 | GK | 12 | 28 | 22 | 17 | 94 |
| Sheehan 2000 | GK | 43 | 44 | 20 | 63 | 100 |
| Hoybye 2001 | LINAC | 18 | 204 | --- | 83 | 83 |
| Kobayashi 2003 | --- | 20 | 64 | 29 | 35 | 100 |
| Devin 2004 | GK | 35 | 42 | 15 | 49 | 91 |
| Castinetti 2007 | GK | 40 | 55 | 29.5 | 42 | 100 |
| Jagannathan 2007 | GK | 90 | 45 | 25 | 42 | 100 |
| Brau 2011* | LINAC | 10 | 50 | 20.7 | 40 | 90 |

Table 4. Summary of cases involving Radiosurgery in patients with Cushing's disease. (*Unpublished manuscript in writing)

Jagannathan et al., 2007; Kobayashi et al., 2002; Morange-Ramos et al., 1998; Petrovich et al., 2003; Witt et al., 1998). In series with at least ten patients and a median follow-up of 2 years, endocrine remission rates range from 17% to 83% (Kobayashi et al., 2002; Mahmoud-Ahmed & Suh, 2002; Morange-Ramos et al., 1998, Petrovich et al., 2003). Rähn and associates (Flickenger et al., 1992) reported their experience at the Karolinska Institute involving 59 patients with Cushing's disease who were treated using the Gamma Knife and followed for 2–15 years. The efficacy rate of the initial treatment was 50%, with retreatment eventually providing normalization of cortisol production in 76% of patients (Rahn et al, 1980).

### 7.2.3 Prolactin-secreting adenomas

We use radiosurgery as a treatment for prolactinomas after failure of medical and/or surgical treatment. Ideally most of the prolactinomas should be treated with medication. Prolactinomas tumor control with medications has been reported around 80-90% (Ferone et al., 2007). Despite having good control, some patients do not tolerate the medications due to side effects and other turnout to be allergic to it.

In our series two patients were treated as primary therapy for medical reasons. Most of the patients were treated following microsurgery. Of the seven patients treated at our institution, complete normalization of prolactin levels occurred in only 14.2%, at an average time of 22 months, with a mean prescription dose of 18.7Gy. Tumor control was achieved in 100% of the cases, but did not correlate with hormone remission.

In published studies of radiosurgery for prolactinomas, the mean prescription dose has varied from 13.3 Gy to 33 Gy, and remission rates varied from 0% to 84% (Table 5) (Kim et al., 1999, 2007; Landolt & Lomax, 2000; Laws & Vance, 1999; Post & Habas, 1990; Pouratian et al., 2006; Yildiz et al., 1999). Variations in success rate are likely related to the dose delivered to the tumor as well as other factors. Witt et al. noted no remissions with a prescription dose of 19 Gy (Witt et al., 1998; Witt, 2003). Pan et al. (Pan et al., 2000) reported a 52% endocrine "cure" rate in a retrospective study of 128 patients in whom GKRS was used as first-line treatment for prolactinomas with a prescription dose of 30 Gy. This study is on a large sample size, and is interesting in that GKRS was used as a first-line treatment before medical therapy.

| Author and Year | RSx Unit | Pt No | F/U (mos) | Peripheral Dose (Gy) | Hormone Normalization (%) | Tumor Control (%) |
|---|---|---|---|---|---|---|
| Mitsumori 1998 | LINAC | 4 | 47 | 15 | 0 | 100 |
| Yoon 1998 | LINAC | 11 | 49 | 17 | 84 | 96 |
| Mokry 1999 | GK | 21 | 31 | 14 | 21 | NR |
| Pan 2000 | GK | 128 | 33 | 31.5 | 52 | 98.4 |
| Choi 2003 | GK | 21 | 42.5 | 28.5 | 24 | 100 |
| Muramatsu 2003 | LINAC | 1 | 30 | 15 | 0 | 100 |
| Pouratian 2006 | GK | 23 | 58 | 18.6 | 24 | 89 |
| Brau 2011* | LINAC | 7 | 35.7 | 18.7 | 14.2 | 100 |

Table 5. Summary of cases involving Radiosurgery in patients with prolactinomas.
(*Unpublished manuscript in writing)

### 7.2.4 Nelson's syndrome

Compared with nonfunctioning and other functioning pituitary adenomas, much less information is available about the efficacy of stereotactic radiosurgery for the treatment of Nelson syndrome. A subset of Cushing's patients do not achieve hormone normalization following microsurgery and radiosurgery, and undergo adrenalectomy as a "salvage" treatment for their disease. Although adrenalectomy is the definitive treatment for cortisol overproduction, a subset of patients may develop Nelson's syndrome, characterized by rapid adenoma growth, hyper-pigmentation and tumor invasion into the parasellar structures (Nagesser et al., 2000). This is thought to be related to the lack of feedback on the hypothalamus and the pituitary gland by the lack of cortisol.

| Author and Year | RSx Unit | Pt No | F/U (mos) | Peripheral Dose (Gy) | Hormone Normalization (%) | Tumor Control (%) |
|---|---|---|---|---|---|---|
| Ganz 1993 | GKS | 3 | 18 | NR | 0 | 100 |
| Wolffenbuttel 1998 | GKS | 1 | 33 | 12 | 0 | 100 |
| Kobayashi 2002 | GKS | 6 | 63 | 28.7 | 33 | 100 |
| Pollock 2002 | GKS | 11 | 37 | 20 | 24 | 82 |
| Vogues 2006 | LINAC | 9 | 63/47a | 15.3 | 16.7 | 89 |
| Mauerman 2007 | GKS | 23 | 20/50a | 25 | 17/60b | 91 |

Table 6. Endocrine and radiographic outcomes of GKRS for Nelson's syndrome. (a) Mean imaging follow-up/mean endocrine follow-up (b)ACTH levels decreased/ACTH reduced to normal values (50 pg/ml)

Pollock and Young reported on 11 patients who underwent GKRS for Nelson's syndrome. They reported control of tumor growth in 9 of 11 patients, with ACTH normalization in four patients (36%) (Pollock & Young, 2002).

There are relatively few studies detailing the results of radiosurgery for Nelson's syndrome (Table 6) ( Ganz, 2000; Ganz et al., 1993; Kobayashi et al., 2002; Laws & Vance, 1999; Levy et al., 1991; Mauermann et al., 2007; Pollock & Wolffenbuttel et al., 1998; Young, 2002). These studies report a mean tumor dose from between 12 Gy to 28.7 Gy, and an endocrine remission rate ranging from 0% to 36%, although only a minority of these studies defined what was meant by endocrine remission. Even cases where endocrine remission was not achieved, tumor growth control rates were favorable, ranging from 82% to 100%.

## 8. Complications following radiosurgery for pituitary adenomas

As previously stated, the most common problem after radiosurgery is development of hypopituitarism. Several groups have reported a low incidence (0-36%) of pituitary dysfunction following radiosurgery (Jagannathan et al., 2007; Jane et al., 2003; Sheehan et al., 2006; Pollock et al., 1994). This incidence is likely higher when patients are followed long-term, with the Karolinska Institute reporting a 72% incidence of hypopituitarism when patients were followed over 10 years (Hoybye et al., 2001). We have observed an overall risk of 20-30% for development of new hormone deficiency following radiosurgery without a significant difference across tumor pathologies. Recent studies using the Cyberknife for secretory adenomas, points to a significantly lower (9.5%) rate of endocrinopathy, although these studies are limited by follow-up of 12 months and less in some cases (Adler et al., 2006; Kajiwara et al., 2005; Pham et al., 2004).

Ultimately, total dose prescribed and the prescription (margin) doses are likely the major factors determining the risk and onset of radiation induced hypopituitarism. The sequence of hormone loss following pituitary radiosurgery is unknown. The difficulty with determining the exact incidence of radiosurgery-induced hypopituitarism stems in part from the fact that many of the patients have previously undergone resection and some fractionated radiotherapy. In addition, pituitary deficiencies may results in part from aging. Thus, it is likely that hypopituitarism in the post-radiosurgical population is multifactorial in cause and related to radiosurgery as well as age-related changes and previous treatments (for example, microsurgery and radiotherapy). In spite of this, however, some have argued that the GH axis is the most sensitive to the late effects of radiation, with the radiation induced defect likely occurring at the hypothalamic level (Blacklay et al., 1986; Shalet, 1993). The gonadotropin and corticotrophin axes are also thought to be sensitive to radiation damage. Diabetes insipidus appears to be uncommon after radiosurgery with only sporadic case reports (Piedra et al., 2004). A well-controlled, long-term study focusing on this issue is needed to determine definitively the incidence of radiosurgery-induced hypopituitarism.

Cranial neuropathies following radiosurgery are exceedingly rare following the first procedure, although the incidence may increase on re-treatment (Jagannathan et al., 2007). Visual injury in general can be avoided if the dose to the optic apparatus is restricted to less than 8 Gy (see previous discussion).

Injury to the cavernous segment of the carotid artery or brain parenchyma is uncommon following radiosurgery. Pollock and associates have recommended that the prescription dose should be limited to less than 50% of the intracavernous CA vessel diameter (Pollock & Carpenter, 2003). Shin recommended restricting the dose to the internal CA to less than 30 Gy (Shin et al., 2000).

Parenchymal brain injury can be present especially in the hypothalamic and temporal regions. Patients with injuries to medial temporal lobes can present with complex partial seizures or if the injury is bilateral with recent memory impairment. Induction of cavernous malformations following radiosurgery to the sellar region is also theoretically possible but thus far has not been reported.

The exact incidence of radiosurgical-induced neoplasm is unknown at present, although we have not seen one in our series of pituitary patients treated with m-LINAC system. Loeffler and colleagues recently reported on 6 patients, including 2 patients with pituitary adenomas who developed new tumors following radiosurgery (Loeffler et al., 2003). They concluded that although the risk of new tumor formation after radiosurgery appears to be significantly less than that seen following fractionated radiotherapy, new tumors can develop in the full dose region as well as in the low-dose periphery of the radiosurgical field. The latency to new tumor formation in this small series (between 6 years and 20 years) was similar to that seen after conventional radiation therapy.

## 9. Prognosis and follow-up

Prognosis for pituitary adenoma patients is largely dependent upon the adenoma size and functionality as well as the patients' pre-radiosurgical status. Patients being treated for pituitary adenomas must be followed long-term with serial clinical, ophthalmological, endocrine and radiological evaluations.

Serial visual field examinations and hormonal screening should be performed. In the majority of cases serial testing of adrenal, thyroid function and GH reserves may be required as well. Patients receiving hormone replacement should have their replacement therapy adjusted as necessary.

Finally, serial MR imaging should be performed to assess for tumor recurrence. It is our practice to perform an initial post-radiosurgical MRI at 6 months after treatment with follow-up MRI's yearly thereafter, unless otherwise indicated. Endocrine and ophthalmologic follow-up should typically occur at the same time to provide adequate correlation with the treatment. There should be a good communication with every discipline involved in the treatment of these patients.

## 10. Conclusions

Multimodality treatment is often used to manage pituitary adenomas. Therapeutic options include medical management, microsurgery, radiosurgery, and radiotherapy. Except for prolactinomas, microsurgery remains the primary treatment for sellar lesions in surgically fit patients, particularly when the lesion is exerting a mass effect on the optic apparatus or producing hormone overproduction. Nevertheless, 20 to 50% of patients experience recurrence of their adenomas, and adjuvant treatment is recommended for these patients.

Stereotactic radiosurgery has been demonstrated to be a safe and highly effective treatment for patients with recurrent or residual pituitary adenomas. Radiosurgery affords effective growth control and hormone normalization for patients and has a generally shorter latency period than that of fractionated radiotherapy. This shorter latency period with radiosurgery can typically be managed with hormone-suppressive medications. Furthermore, the complications (for example, radiation-induced neoplasia and cerebral vasculopathy) associated with radiosurgery appear to occur less frequently than those associated with radiotherapy. Radiosurgery may even serve as a primary treatment for those patients deemed unfit for microsurgical tumor removal because they have other co morbidities or demonstrable tumors in a surgically inaccessible location. Radiosurgery can frequently preserve and, at times, even restore neurological and hormone function.

Radiosurgery is a useful tool in the treatment of both secretory and non-secretory pituitary adenomas. In most patients, radiosurgery controls adenoma growth. However, normalization of hormone overproduction can vary considerably depending on the patients' presenting condition. Challenges for the future include delineating the optimal timing for the administration of antisecretory medications and identifying factors that can improve the response of pituitary adenomas to radiosurgery. Finally, physicians caring for patients with pituitary disorders should establish uniform endocrinological criteria and diagnostic testing for pre- and post-radiosurgical evaluations.

## 11. References

Abe T, Yamamoto M, Taniyama M, Tanioka D, Izumiyama H, Matsumoto K (2002) Early palliation of oculomotor nerve palsy following gamma knife radiosurgery for pituitary adenoma. *Eur Neurol* 47:61–63.

Adler JR Jr, Chang SD, Murphy MJ, Doty J, Geis P, Hancock SL (1997) The Cyberknife: a frameless robotic system for radiosurgery. *Funct Neurosurg* 69: 124-128.

Adler JR Jr, Gibbs IC, Puataweepong P, Chang SD (2006) Visual field preservation after multisession cyberknife radiosurgery for perioptic lesions. *Neurosurgery* 59:244-254 discussion 244-254

Arnaldi G, Angeli A, Atkinson AB, Bertagna X, Cavagnini F, Chrousos GP, Fava GA, Findling JW, Gaillard RC, Grossman AB, Kola B, Lacroix A, Mancini T, Mantero F, Newell-Price J, Nieman LK, Sonino N, Vance ML, Giustina A, Boscaro M (2003) Diagnosis and complications of Cushing's syndrome: a consensus statement. J *Clin Endocrinol Metab* 88:5593-5602.

Becker, G., Kocher, M., Kortmann, R.D., Paulsen, F., Jeremic, B., Muller, R.P. & Bamberg, M. (2002) Radiation therapy in the multimodal treatment approach of pituitary adenoma. *Strahlentherapie und Onkologie*, 178, 173-186.

Blacklay A, Grossman A, Ross RJ, Savage MO, Davies PS, Plowman PN, Coy DH, Besser GM (1986) Cranial irradiation for cerebral and nasopharyngeal tumors in children: evidence for the production of a hypothalamic defect in growth hormone release. *J Endocrinol* 108:25-29

Brada, M., Burchell, L., Ashley, S. & Traish, D. (1999) The incidence of cerebrovascular accidents in patients with pituitary adenoma. *International Journal of Radiation Oncology, Biology, Physics*, 45, 693-698.

Brada, M., Ford, D., Ashley, S., Bliss, J.M., Crowley, S., Mason, M., Rajan, B. & Traish, D. (1992) Risk of second brain tumor after conservative surgery and radiotherapy for pituitary adenoma. *British Medical Journal*, 304, 1343-1346.

Brada, M., Rajan, B., Traish, D., Ashley, S., Holmes-Sellors, P.J., Nussey, S. & Utley, D. (1993) The long-term efficacy of conservative surgery and radiotherapy in the control of pituitary adenomas. *Clinical Endocrinology*, 38, 571-578.

Brada, M., Ashley, S., Ford, D., Traish, D., Burchell, L. & Rajan, B. (2002) Cerebrovascular mortality in patients with pituitary adenoma. *Clinical Endocrinology*, 57, 713-717.

Buchfelder M, Fahlbusch R, Schott W, Honegger J (1991) Long term follow-up results in hormonally active pituitary adenomas after primary successful transsphenoidal surgery. *Acta Neurochir Suppl (Wien)* 53:72-76

Chang SD, Murphy M, Geis P, Martin DP, Hancock SL, Doty JR, Adler JR Jr (1998) Clinical experience with image-guided robotic radiosurgery (the Cyberknife) in the treatment of brain and spinal cord tumors. *Neurol Med Chir* 38:780-783.

Chen JC, Giannotta SL, Yu C, Petrovich Z, Levy ML, Apuzzo ML (2001) Radiosurgical management of benign cavernous sinus tumors: dose profiles and acute complications. *Neurosurgery* 48:1022-1030 discussion 1030-1022

Chen JC, Giannotta SL, Yu C, Petrovich Z, Levy ML, Apuzzo ML (2001) Radiosurgical management of benign cavernous sinus tumors: dose profiles and acute complications. *Neurosurgery* 48:1022-1030 discussion 1030-1022

Chu JW, Matthias DF, Belanoff J, Schatzberg A, Hoffman AR, Feldman D (2001) Successful long-term treatment of refractory Cushing's disease with high-dose mifepristone (RU 486). J *Clin Endocrinol Metab* 86:3568-3573.

Ciric I, Ragin A, Baumgartner C, Pierce D (1997) Complications of transsphenoidal surgery: results of a national survey, review of the literature, and personal experience. *Neurosurgery* 40:225-236 discussion 236-227

Cozzi R, Barausse M, Asnaghi D, Dallabonzana D, Lodrini S, Attanasio R (2001) Failure of radiotherapy in acromegaly. *Eur J Endocrinol* 145:717–726.

Erfurth, E.M., Bulow, B., Mikoczy, Z., Svahn-Tapper, G. & Hagmar, L. (2001) Is there an increase in second brain tumours after surgery and irradiation for a pituitary tumour? *Clinical Endocrinology*, 55, 613–616.

Erfurth, E.M., Bulow, B., Svahn-Tapper, G., Norrving, B., Odh, K., Mikoczy, Z., Bjork, J. & Hagmar, L. (2002) Risk factors for cerebrovascular deaths in patients operated and irradiated for pituitary tumors. *Journal of Clinical Endocrinology and Metabolism*, 87, 4892–4899.

Feigl GC, Bonelli CM, Berghold A, Mokry M (2002) Effects of gamma knife radiosurgery of pituitary adenomas on pituitary function. *J Neurosurg* 97:415–421

Ferone D, Pivonello R, Resmini E, Boschetti M, Rebora A, Albertelli M, Albanese V, Colao A, Culler MD, Minuto F. Preclinical and clinical experiences with the role of dopamine receptors in the treatment of pituitary adenomas. *Eur J Endocrinol*. 2007 Apr; 156 Suppl 1:S37-43.

Flickinger JC, Lunsford LD, Kondziolka D (1992) Dose prescription and dose-volume effects in radiosurgery. *Neurosurg Clin N Am* 3:51–59

Freda PU (2003) How effective are current therapies for acromegaly? *Growth Horm IGF Res* 13(Suppl A): S144–S151

Fukuoka S, Ito T, Takanashi M, Hojo A, Nakamura H (2001) Gamma knife radiosurgery for growth hormone-secreting pituitary adenomas invading the cavernous sinus. *Stereotact Funct Neurosurg* 76:213–217.

Ganz JC (2002) Gamma knife radiosurgery and its possible relationship to malignancy: a review. *J Neurosurg* 97:644–652

Ganz JC, Backlund EO, Thorsen FA (1993) The effects of Gamma Knife surgery of pituitary adenomas on tumor growth and endocrinopathies. *Stereotact Funct Neurosurg* 61(Suppl 1):30–37.

Giustina A, Barkan A, Casanueva FF, Cavagnini F, Frohman L, Ho K, Veldhuis J, Wass J, Von Werder K, Melmed S (2000) Criteria for cure of acromegaly: a consensus statement. *J Clin Endocrinol Metab* 85:526–529

Hayashi M, Izawa M, Hiyama H, Nakamura S, Atsuchi S, Sato H, et al: Gamma knife radiosurgery for pituitary adenomas. *Stereotact Funct Neurosurg* 72 (Suppl 1):111-118, 1999

Hayashi M, Taira T, Ochiai T, Chernov M, Takasu Y, Izawa M, Kouyama N, Tomida M, Tokumaru O, Katayama Y, Kawakami Y, Hori T, Takakura K (2005) Gamma knife surgery of the pituitary: new treatment for thalamic pain syndrome. *J Neurosurg* 102:38–41 Suppl

Horvath E, Kovacs K, Scheithauer BW, Randall RV, Laws ER Jr, Thorner MO, Tindall GT, Barrow DL (1983) Pituitary adenomas producing growth hormone, prolactin, and one or more glycoprotein hormones: a histologic, immunohistochemical, and ultrastructural study of four surgically removed tumors. *Ultrastruct Pathol* 5:171-183.

Hoybye C, Grenback E, Rahn T, Degerblad M, Thoren M, Hulting AL (2001) Adrenocorticotropic hormone-producing pituitary tumors: 12- to 22-year follow-up after treatment with stereotactic radiosurgery. *Neurosurgery* 49:284–291 discussion 291–282

Ikeda H, Jokura H, Yoshimoto T (2001) Transsphenoidal surgery and adjuvant gamma knife treatment for growth hormone-secreting pituitary adenoma. *J Neurosurg* 95:285–291

Izawa M, Hayashi M, Nakaya K, Satoh H, Ochiai T, Hori T, Takakura K (2000) Gamma knife radiosurgery for pituitary adenomas. *J Neurosurg* 93(Suppl 3):19–22

Jackson IM, Noren G (1999) Gamma knife radiosurgery for pituitary tumors. *Best Pract Res Clin Endocrinol Metab* 13:461–469.

Jagannathan J, Dumont AS, Jane JA Jr, Laws ER Jr (2005) Pediatric sellar tumors: diagnostic procedures and management. *Neurosurg Focus* 18:6.

Jagannathan J, Sheehan JP, Pouratian N, Laws ER, Steiner L, Vance ML (2007) Gamma knife surgery for Cushing's disease. *J Neurosurg* 106:980–987.

Jane JA Jr, Vance ML, Woodburn CJ, Laws ER Jr (2003) Stereotactic radiosurgery for hypersecreting pituitary tumors: part of a multimodality approach. *Neurosurg Focus* 14:e12.

Jezkova J, Marek J, Hana V, Krsek M, Weiss V, Vladyka V, Lisak R, Vymazal J, Pecen L (2006) Gamma knife Radiosurgery for acromegaly - long-term experience. *Clin Endocrinol* 64:588–595.

Kajiwara K, Saito K, Yoshikawa K, Kato S, Akimura T, Nomura S, Ishihara H, Suzuki M (2005) Image-guided stereotactic radiosurgery with the CyberKnife for pituitary adenomas. *Minim Invasive Neurosurg* 48:91–96.

Kajiwara K, Saito K, Yoshikawa K, Kato S, Akimura T, Nomura S, Ishihara H, Suzuki M (2005) Image-guided stereotactic radiosurgery with the CyberKnife for pituitary adenomas. *Minim Invasive Neurosurg* 48:91–96.

Kanter AS, Diallo AO, Jane JA Jr, Sheehan JP, Asthagiri AR, Oskouian RJ, Okonkwo DO, Sansur CA, Vance ML, Rogol AD, Laws ER Jr (2005) Single-center experience with pediatric Cushing's disease. *J Neurosurg* 103:413–420

Kim MS, Lee SI, Sim JH (1999) Gamma Knife radiosurgery for functioning pituitary microadenoma. *Stereotact Funct Neurosurg* 72(Suppl 1):119–124.

Kim SH, Huh R, Chang JW, Park YG, Chung SS (1999) Gamma Knife radiosurgery for functioning pituitary adenomas. *Stereotact Funct Neurosurg* 72(Suppl 1):101–110.

Kobayashi T, Kida Y, Mori Y (2002) Gamma knife Radiosurgery in the treatment of Cushing disease: long-term results. *J Neurosurg* 97:422–428

Landolt AM, Haller D, Lomax N, Scheib S, Schubiger O, Siegfried J, Wellis G (2000) Octreotide may act as a radio protective agent in acromegaly. *J Clin Endocrinol Metab* 85:1287–1289.

Landolt AM, Haller D, Lomax N, Scheib S, Schubiger O, Siegfried J, Wellis G (1998) Stereotactic radiosurgery for recurrent surgically treated acromegaly: comparison with fractionated radiotherapy. *J Neurosurg* 88:1002–1008

Landolt AM, Lomax N (2000) Gamma knife radiosurgery for prolactinomas. J Neurosurg 93(Suppl 3):14–18.

Laws ER Jr, Ebersold MJ, Piepgras DG, Randall RV, Salassa RM (1985) The results of transsphenoidal surgery in specific clinical entities. In: *Management of pituitary adenomas and related lesions with emphasis on Transsphenoidal microsurgery.* Laws ER Jr, Randall RV, Kern EB et al (eds) Appleton-Century-Crofts, New York, pp 277-305

Laws ER Jr, Fode NC, Redmond MJ (1985) Transsphenoidalsurgery following unsuccessful prior therapy. An assessment of benefits and risks in 158 patients. *J Neurosurg* 63:823–829

Laws ER Jr, Thapar K (1996) Recurrent pituitary adenomas. In: *Pituitary adenomas.* Landolt AM, Vance ML, Reilly PL (eds) Churchill-Livingtone, Edinburgh, pp 385-394

Laws ER Jr, Vance ML (1999) Radiosurgery for pituitary tumors and craniopharyngiomas. *Neurosurg Clin N Am* 10:327–336

Laws ER, Sheehan JP (2006) Pituitary surgery: a modern approach. *Front Horm Res.* Basel, Karger vol 34, pp I-X

Laws ER, Vance ML, Thapar K (2000) Pituitary surgery for the management of acromegaly. *Horm Res* 53(Suppl 3):71–75.

Leber KA, Bergloff J, Langmann G, Mokry M, Schrottner O, Pendl G (1995) Radiation sensitivity of visual and oculomotor pathways. *Stereotact Funct Neurosurg* 64(Suppl 1):233–238

Leber KA, Bergloff J, Pendl G (1998) Dose-response tolerance of the visual pathways and cranial nerves of the cavernous sinus to stereotactic radiosurgery. *J Neurosurg* 88:43–50.

Levy RP, Fabrikant JI, Frankel KA, Phillips MH, Lyman JT, Lawrence JH, Tobias CA (1991) Heavy-charged-particle Radiosurgery of the pituitary gland: clinical results of 840 patients. *Stereotact Funct Neurosurg* 57:22–35.

Lim YL, Leem W, Kim TS, Rhee BA, Kim GK (1998) Four years' experiences in the treatment of pituitary adenomas with gamma knife radiosurgery. *Stereotact Funct Neurosurg* 70(Suppl1):95–109.

Loeffler JS, Niemierko A, Chapman PH (2003) Second tumors after radiosurgery: tip of the iceberg or a bump in the road? *Neurosurgery* 52:1436–1440 discussion 1440–1432

Losa M, Valle M, Mortini P, Franzin A, Da Passano CF, Cenzato M, et al. (2004) Gamma Knife surgery for treatment of residual nonfunctioning pituitary adenomas after surgical debulking. *J Neurosurg* 100:438–444

Mahmoud-Ahmed AS, Suh JH (2002) Radiation therapy for Cushing's disease: a review. *Pituitary* 5:175–180.

Mampalam TJ, Tyrrell JB, Wilson CB (1988) Transsphenoidal microsurgery for Cushing disease. A report of 216 cases. *Ann Intern Med* 109:487–493

Mauermann WJ, Sheehan JP, Chernavvsky DR, Laws ER, Steiner L, Vance ML (2007) Gamma Knife surgery for adrenocorticotropic hormone-producing pituitary adenomas after bilateral adrenalectomy. *J Neurosurg* 106:988–993.

Mitsumori M, Shrieve DC, Alexander E III, Kaiser UB, Richardson GE, Black PM, et al. (1998): Initial clinical results of LINAC-based stereotactic radiosurgery and stereotactic radiotherapy for pituitary adenomas. *Int J Radiat Oncol Biol Phys* 42:573–580

Mokry M, Ramschak-Schwarzer S, Simbrunner J, Ganz JC, Pendl G (1999): A six year experience with the postoperative radiosurgical management of pituitary adenomas. *Stereotact Funct Neurosurg* 72 (Suppl 1):88–100

Morange-Ramos I, Regis J, Dufour H, Andrieu JM, Grisoli F, Jaquet P, Peragut JC (1998) Gamma-knife surgery for secreting pituitary adenomas. *Acta Neurochir* (Wien) 140:437–443.

Muramatsu J, Yoshida M, Shioura H, Kawamura Y, Ito H, Takeuchi H, et al. (2003): [Clinical results of LINAC-based stereotactic Radiosurgery for pituitary adenoma.] *Nippon Igaku Hoshasen Gakkai Zasshi* 63:225–230

Nagesser SK, van Seters AP, Kievit J, Hermans J, Krans HM, van de Velde CJ (2000) Long-term results of total adrenalectomy for Cushing's disease. *World J Surg* 24:108–113.

Nieman LK (2002) Medical therapy of Cushing's disease. Pituitary 5:77–82.

Pan L, Zhang N, Wang EM, Wang BJ, Dai JZ, Cai PW (2000) Gamma knife radiosurgery as a primary treatment for prolactinomas. *J Neurosurg* 93(Suppl 3):10–13

Petrovich Z, Yu C, Giannotta SL, Zee CS, Apuzzo ML (2003) Gamma knife radiosurgery for pituitary adenoma: early results. *Neurosurgery* 53:51–59 discussion 59–61

Pham CJ, Chang SD, Gibbs IC, Jones P, Heilbrun MP, Adler JR Jr (2004) Preliminary visual field preservation after staged CyberKnife radiosurgery for perioptic lesions. *Neurosurgery* 54:799–810 discussion 810 812

Piedra MP, Brown PD, Carpenter PC, Link MJ (2004) Resolution of diabetes insipidus following gamma knife surgery for a solitary metastasis to the pituitary stalk. Case report. *J Neurosurg* 101:1053–1056

Pollock BE, Carpenter PC: Stereotactic radiosurgery as an alternative to fractionated radiotherapy for patients with recurrent or residual nonfunctioning pituitary adenomas. *Neurosurgery* 53: 1086–1094, 2003

Pollock BE, Cochran J, Nat N, Brown PD, Erickson D, Link MJ, Garces YI, Foote RL, Stafford SL, Shomberg PJ. (2008) Gamma knife Radiosurgery for patients with nonfunctioning pituitary adenomas: results from a 15 year experience. *Int J Radiat Oncol Biol Phys*. 70(5): 1325-9.

Pollock BE, Jacob JT, Brown PD, Nippoldt TB (2007) Radiosurgery of growth hormone-producing pituitary adenomas: factors associated with biochemical remission. *J Neurosurg* 106:833–838.

Pollock BE, Kondziolka D, Lunsford LD, Flickinger JC (1994) Stereotactic radiosurgery for pituitary adenomas: imaging, visual and endocrine results. *Acta Neurochir Suppl* (Wien) 62:33–38

Pollock BE, Young WF Jr (2002) Stereotactic radiosurgery for patients with ACTH-producing pituitary adenomas after prior adrenalectomy. *Int J Radiat Oncol Biol Phys* 54:839–841.

Post KD, Habas JE (1990) Comparison of long term results between prolactin secreting adenomas and ACTH secreting adenomas. *Can J Neurol Sci* 17:74–77

Pouratian N, Sheehan J, Jagannathan J, Laws ER Jr, Steiner L, Vance ML (2006) Gamma knife radiosurgery for medically and surgically refractory prolactinomas. *Neurosurgery* 59:255–266 discussion 255–266.

Rahn T, Thoren M, Hall K, Backlund EO (1980) Stereotactic radiosurgery in Cushing's syndrome: acute radiation effects. *Surg Neurol* 14:85–92

Shalet SM (1993) Radiation and pituitary dysfunction. *N Engl J Med* 328:131–133.

Sheehan JM, Vance ML, Sheehan JP, Ellegala DB, Laws ER Jr (2000) Radiosurgery for Cushing's disease after failed transsphenoidal surgery. *J Neurosurg* 93:738–742

Sheehan JP, Jagannathan J, Pouratian N, Steiner L (2006) Stereotactic radiosurgery for pituitary adenomas: a review of the literature and our experience. *Front Horm Res* 34:185–205

Sheehan JP, Kondziolka D, Flickinger J, Lunsford LD (2002) Radiosurgery for residual or recurrent nonfunctioning pituitary adenoma. J Neurosurg 97:408–414

Sheehan JP, Kondziolka D, Flickinger J, Lunsford LD (2002): Radiosurgery for residual or recurrent nonfunctioning pituitary adenoma. *J Neurosurg* 97 (Suppl 5):408–414

Shin M, Kurita H, Sasaki T, Tago M, Morita A, Ueki K, Kirino T (2000) Stereotactic radiosurgery for pituitary adenoma invading the cavernous sinus. *J Neurosurg* 93(Suppl 3):2–5

Tomlinson, J.W., Holden, N., Hills, R.K., Wheatley, K., Clayton, R.N., Bates, A.S., Sheppard, M.C. & Stewart, P.M. (2001) Association between premature mortality and hypopituitarism. West Midlands Prospective Hypopituitary Study Group. *Lancet*, 357, 425–431.

Tsang, R.W., Brierley, J.D., Panzarella, T., Gospodarowicz, M.K., Sutcliffe, S.B. & Simpson, W.J. (1994) Radiation therapy for pituitary adenoma: treatment outcome and prognostic factors. *International Journal of Radiation Oncology, Biology, Physics*, 30, 557–565

Vance ML (1998) Endocrinological evaluation of acromegaly. *J Neurosurg* 89:499–500

Witt TC (2003) Stereotactic radiosurgery for pituitary tumors. *Neurosurg Focus* 14:e10.

Witt TC, Kondziolka D, Flickinger JC, Lunsford LD (1998) Gamma knife radiosurgery for pituitary tumors. In: *Gamma knife brain surgery progress in neurological surgery.* Lunsford LD, Kondziolka D, Flickinger J (eds) Karger, Basel, pp114–127.

Wolffenbuttel BH, Kitz K, Beuls EM (1998) Beneficial gammaknife radiosurgery in a patient with Nelson's syndrome. *Clin Neurol Neurosurg* 100:60–63.

Wowra B, Stummer W (2002) Efficacy of gamma knife Radiosurgery for nonfunctioning pituitary adenomas: a quantitative follow up with magnetic resonance imaging-based volumetric analysis. *J Neurosurg* 97:429–432

Yildiz F, Zorlu F, Erbas T, Atahan L (1999) Radiotherapy in the management of giant pituitary adenomas. *Radiother Oncol* 52:233–237.

Yoon SC, Suh TS, Jang HS, Chung SM, Kim YS, Ryu MR, et al. 1998 Clinical results of 24 pituitary macroadenomas with linac based stereotactic radiosurgery. *Int J Radiat Onc Biol Phys* 41:849–853